OSTEOF

All the advice you need for preventing bone loss

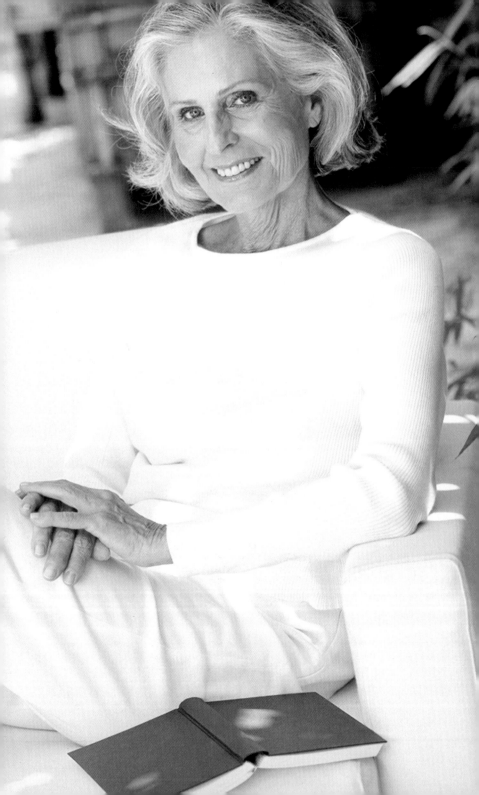

OSTEOPOROSIS

All the advice you need for preventing bone loss

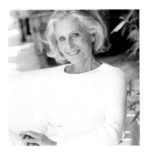

Dr Gabrielle Cremer
Aurélie Ober

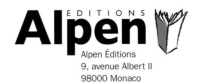

EDITIONS
Alpen

Alpen Éditions
9, avenue Albert II
98000 Monaco

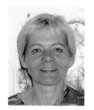

Dr Gabrielle Cremer is a clinical pharmacologist, and has worked in the pharmaceutical industry for several years. She has run a medical communications company in Strasbourg since 2005 and works in three languages. She has written many scientific publications. For more information, please see the website www.cremerconsulting.com

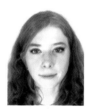

Aurelie Ober has a Master's degree in translation. Since completing her studies she has worked exclusively in the area of medicine and regularly publishes medical articles for the greater public. Her working languages are French, English, and German.

Exclusive copyrights:
© Alpen Éditions
9, avenue Albert II
MC - 98000 MONACO
Tel: 00377 97 77 62 10
Fax: 00377 97 77 62 11
Web: www.alpen.mc

Managing Publisher: Christophe Didierlaurent
Editorial: Fabienne Desmarets and Sandra Del Barba
Designer: Stéphane Falaschi

Copyrights:
Banana Stock, BrandX, Digital vision, Fancy, Image State, Pixtal, Stockbyte, Thinkstock

ISBN13: 978-2-35934-063-1

Printed in Italy

Introduction

Osteoporosis is a widespread condition that affects both individuals and society as a whole. But what exactly is osteoporosis? According to the World Health Organization, osteoporosis is defined as a loss in bone mass and a deterioration of the bone microarchitecture, which makes the bones brittle, fragile, and prone to fractures.

In both men and women, bone mass reaches a peak around the age of 20 years. Bone mass depends not only on genetic factors, but also on diet, particularly the intake of calcium and vitamin D, and physical exercise. Bone mass acquired during childhood and adolescence has a major impact on the occurrence of osteoporosis later in life.

Experts recommend that young people consume about 1500mg of calcium per day. However, many studies conducted in the United States have shown that actual calcium intake is far too low. This is a particular problem in young girls, which means that these girls are likely to suffer from osteoporosis later in life. However, it is never too late to change one's lifestyle, and adults must also ensure that they consume enough calcium to maintain the bone mass acquired during adolescence.

For both genders, bone mineral density begins to decrease with age following a peak at about age 20. In women, estrogen somewhat delays this decrease in bone mass until menopause. After menopause, the loss of bone mass increases rapidly, and when this bone

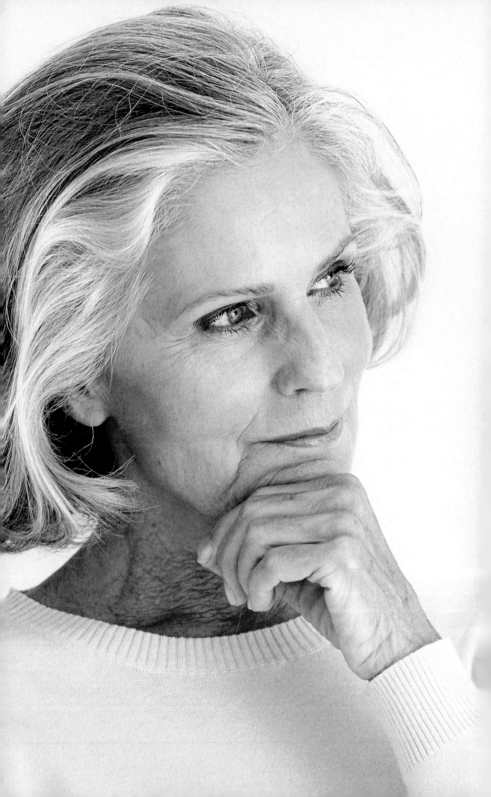

loss reaches a significant level, as assessed by bone densitometry, experts speak of postmenopausal osteoporosis. This type of osteoporosis makes women vulnerable to vertebral compression fractures and wrist fractures. Another form of osteoporosis is known as senile osteoporosis, as it is related to age. This form affects both men and women equally, and makes them susceptible to hip fractures.

This guide aims to help you better understand osteoporosis in order to make appropriate treatment decisions, and better yet, to empower you to make the steps necessary to prevent it. Therefore, our main goal in writing this book is to provide you with clear information so you can better prevent and treat the disease. We hope you enjoy reading our work.

TABLE OF CONTENTS

TABLE OF CONTENTS

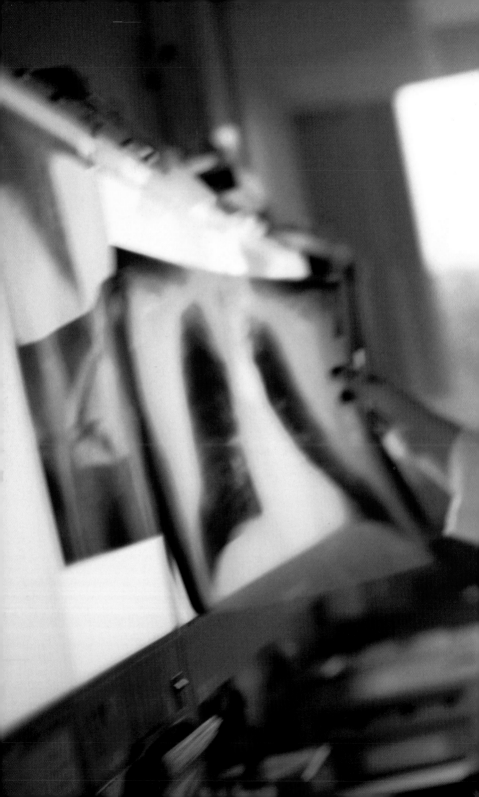

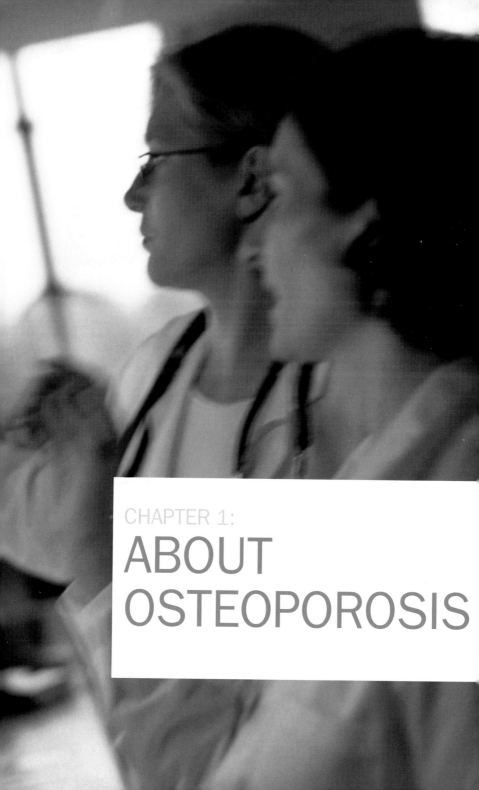

CHAPTER 1:
ABOUT OSTEOPOROSIS

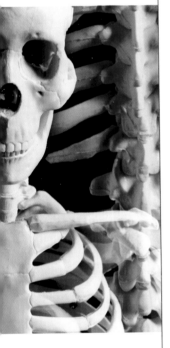

ABOUT OSTEOPOROSIS
Weakened bones

Prior to the use of osteodensitometry in clinical practice, osteoporosis was diagnosed retrospectively, essentially in emergency rooms, in patients admitted for symptomatic fractures. With the advent of new technologies such as osteodensitometry tests, the diagnostic approach to osteoporosis has radically changed. As a result, in 1994, the WHO published a new universal definition of osteoporosis: "Osteoporosis is defined as a systemic skeletal disorder characterized by low bone mass and microarchitectural deterioration of bone tissue, with a consequent increase in bone fragility and susceptibility to fracture."

Low bone density

Osteoporosis is a disease that affects the entire skeleton, in which the overall bone mass is decreased. Currently, bone mass can be precisely determined using highly sophisticated technology known as bone mineral densitometry. This tool allows radiologists to precisely measure bone mineral density (BMD). BMD refers to grams of bone mineral, known as hydroxyapatite, per square centimeter of bone section. A patient's BMD, measured by densitometry and expressed in g/cm^2, is compared with a reference value, which is the mean BMD of young adults of the same gender at their peak bone mass, sometimes referred to as the "young adult mean". When compared with the normal value, a patient's BMD can be expressed in terms of the number of standard deviations (SD) from the normal value. A convenient way to express this is the T-score. The T-score examines a patient's BMD by comparing the amount of actual bone loss with that expected for individuals of the same age and gender.

Bone microarchitecture alterations

In addition to a decreased bone mass, the osteoporotic process also alters bone microarchitecture. During this process, calcium depletes faster than it is replaced, leaving bones thinned, brittle, and prone to injury. This altered bone microarchitecture appears to be an essential diagnostic factor. Currently, many experts suggest that this altered bone microarchitecture should be taken into account when diagnosing osteoporosis, as suggested by the WHO's international guidelines.

Different evolutive stages

The current diagnosis of osteoporosis is based on the results of BMD measurements using DEXA (DEXA=Double Energy X-ray Absorptiometry). According to the WHO

Study Group, the general diagnostic categories with respect to osteoporosis are as follows:
- Normal bone is defined by a bone mineral density (BMD) not more than 1 SD below the young adult mean (T-score above -1).

- Osteopenia, or low bone mass, is defined by a BMD between 1 and 2.5 SD below the young adult mean (T-score between -1 and -2.5). In the case of osteopenia, preventive measures are highly recommended.

- Osteoporosis is defined as a BMD of 2.5 SD or more below the young adult mean . (T-score at or below -2.5).

- Severe osteoporosis or established osteoporosis is defined by a BMD of 2.5 SD or more below the young adult mean in the presence of one or more fragility fractures. In this case, prompt treatment is vital.

Bone osteodensitometry

According to WHO, bone densitometry, also known as DEXA, is the reference technique for diagnosing osteoporosis. By measuring bone mineral density, this technique allows your doctor to diagnose osteoporosis, monitor your condition, and assess the efficacy of different therapeutic measures. Based on the WHO classification system, an individual with a BMD of 2.5 SD or more below the young adult mean suffers from osteoporosis.

A disease related to age and other factors

Osteoporosis can be classified as a primary or secondary condition. Primary osteoporosis is diagnosed when other disorders known to cause osteoporosis have been ruled out. It is the most common type of osteoporosis, occurring mainly in menopausal women or in the elderly. When it occurs in women following menopause, the disease is also referred to as postmenopausal osteoporosis, whereas senile osteoporosis describes the disease occurring in the elderly. Secondary osteoporosis is diagnosed when the condition is related to another illness or to the use of certain drugs.

Primary osteoporosis

Type 1 osteoporosis – postmenopausal osteoporosis – affects postmenopausal women aged 50 to 65 years. Menopause generally occurs around age 50, and marks the end of a woman's childbearing years. Therefore, Type 1 osteoporosis is mainly observed in women with high levels of postmenopausal bone loss and is thought to result primarily from estrogen deficiency caused by menopause. This makes women prone to vertebral compression fractures or wrist fractures should they happen to fall down.

Cushing's syndrome

Cushing's syndrome is a hormonal disorder characterized by obesity, hypertension, and face swelling. This syndrome is caused by body tissues' prolonged exposure to high levels of cortisol secreted by the adrenal glands. It may also be caused by the administration of cortisol-like medications to treat various diseases. The hormone cortisol has a harmful effect on bone mass and thus may contribute to osteoporosis.

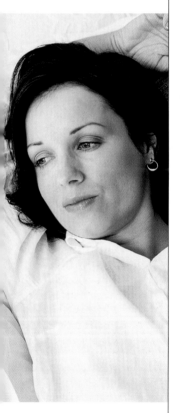

Type 2 osteoporosis or senile osteoporosis is age-related, and mainly affects the elderly after 70 years of age. Bone mass slowly decreases with age, beginning at about age 30. From this age onwards, bone mass decreases approximately 3 to 5% every 10 years. This type of osteoporosis mostly affects the hard outer cortical bone tissue and generally spares the porous spongy bone tissue. Therefore, individuals suffering from senile osteoporosis are prone to hip fractures. Type 3 osteoporosis, or idiopathic juvenile osteoporosis, is a rare disease affecting children aged 8 to 12. Its exact cause is still unknown.

Secondary osteoporosis

Osteoporosis may be secondary to other illnesses such as endocrine disorders. In this context, certain diseases of the thyroid gland or a deficiency in sex hormones, also known as hypogonadism, may lead to the development of secondary osteoporosis. In addition, systemic disorders such as rheumatoid arthritis or idiopathic juvenile arthritis may be responsible for a loss of bone mass. Similarly, certain digestive disorders such as inflammatory bowel diseases or cirrhosis may contribute to secondary osteoporosis.

Osteoporosis may also be related to the use of certain medications. Corticosteroids are likely to induce osteoporosis, if taken in high doses for a prolonged period of time. Furthermore, certain anti-epileptic drugs such as phenytoin or phenobarbital, or anticoagulant drugs such as heparin, have been associated with osteoporosis. Moreover, drugs used to treat hormone-dependant cancers, such as aromatase inhibitors or GnRH agonists, have also been associated with osteoporosis, due to the fact that they suppress hormones.

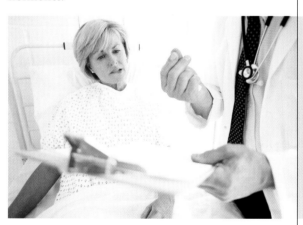

Immobilization osteoporosis

Immobilization due to an accident or certain illnesses may be a major cause of osteoporosis, as it accelerates bone loss. Over a 6-month immobilization period, this bone loss may amount to as much as 40%.

Women and osteoporosis

Men and women are not equal when it comes to osteoporosis. Approximately one out of every three women over 50 suffer from osteoporosis compared with one out of every five men. Over age 80, 70% of all women are affected by osteoporosis. This difference is not merely a coincidence...

Why are women more vulnerable?

The first reason is that bone mass continues to grow for 2 more years in boys as compared to girls, giving males a slight advantage. Towards the end of the growth period, boys have approximately 30% more bone mass than girls.

Testosterone, primarily secreted by the testes in men, is an anabolic hormone that stimulates bone and muscle growth. Men have a higher concentration of testosterone than women, which might explain their lower susceptibility to osteoporosis. Furthermore, the hormonal changes that occur during a woman's life play a deciding role in the occurrence of osteoporosis. Indeed, estrogen plays a significant role in maintaining bone mass in adult women. Therefore, an estrogen deficiency has a direct influence on bone strength.

Menopause, a difficult time

Menopause, which in most women occurs between the ages of 45 and 55, marks a permanent cessation of menstruation, due to a decline in the production of estrogen by the ovaries. In addition to early symptoms such a hot flashes, vaginal dryness, mood changes, weight gain, and sleep disturbances, this decline in estrogen production has a negative effect on bones. During early menopause, bone loss accelerates, and slows down after about 3-5 years. Approximately 30% of postmenopausal women are severely affected by this weakening of the bones and develop osteoporosis.

Premature menopause

Whereas normal menopause usually occurs around the age of 50 years, menopause can occur earlier in some women. This phenomenon, known as premature menopause, affects approximately 1% of women. As in normal menopause, the estrogen deficiency observed during premature menopause accelerates bone loss. Moreover, annual bone loss is higher than in "normal menopausal women", thereby increasing the risk of osteoporosis. This makes premature menopausal women even more prone to fractures of the vertebrae or wrist.

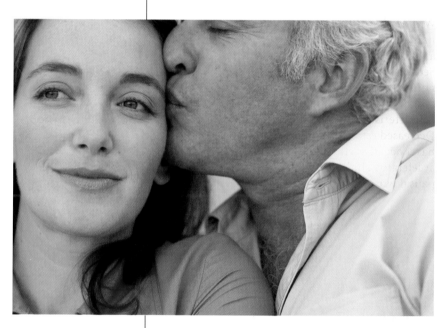

Amenorrhea

Amenorrhea is defined as the absence of menstrual periods occurring in a woman of reproductive age. A girl who does not start menstruating in adolescence is said to have primary amenorrhea. Secondary amenorrhea is more common, and refers to the temporary or permanent cessation of periods in a woman who previously menstruated normally.

While it is common for many women to occasionally miss a period, amenorrhea occurs when a woman misses three or more periods in a row. Secondary amenorrhea may result from anorexia nervosa, which may not only stop menstruation, but may also induce the loss of secondary sex characteristics, such as the breasts or pubic hair. Decreased estrogen production during amenorrhea has a negative effect on bone mass, as bone loss is accelerated similarly to what occurs in postmenopausal women.

Hormone replacement therapy
During and after menopause, a woman's body produces much less estrogen. Hormone replacement therapy may be prescribed to reduce the discomfort of menopausal symptoms such as hot flashes and vaginal dryness. Hormone replacement therapy has also been shown to be effective in the prevention and treatment of osteoporosis, as it reduces bone loss and the associated risk of fractures.

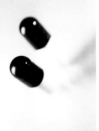

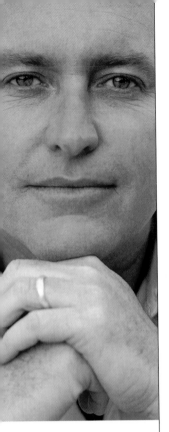

Men and osteoporosis

Osteoporosis is less common in men than in women. Nevertheless, men are still affected by osteoporosis, as approximately 13% of men over age 50 suffer from osteoporotic bone fractures.

Osteoporosis is rarer in men

In 25% of cases, osteoporosis in men leads to hip fractures, generally occurring after age 70.

Several factors may account for this rarer occurrence in men, notably a significantly higher bone density. Unlike women, there is no known hormonal basis for the mid-life transition in men. Thus, in contrast to menopause, which is associated with a sudden decrease in hormone secretion in women, men experience a gradual and very slow decline in testosterone production.

Often another cause is to blame

In about half of all male osteoporosis cases, the cause is unknown. However, several factors are known to contribute to the development of this condition. These causes include testosterone deficiency, also known as hypogonadism.

In addition, excessive alcohol consumption and tobacco use have been associated with osteoporosis in men. Indeed, clinical trials have demonstrated that the risk of vertebral compression fractures is 2.3 times higher in heavy smokers older than 60. In men, the occurrence of osteoporosis may also be linked to digestive disorders, including liver disease. Systemic disorders such as rheumatoid arthritis or ankylosing spondylarthritis have also been associated with the disease. Osteoporosis may also be secondary to thyroid gland dysfunction, such as hyperthyroidism or hyperparathyroidism. Lastly, male osteoporosis may also be linked to hypercalciuria, which refers to excessive calcium concentrations in the urine.

In elderly men, androgen, vitamin D, and calcium deficiencies are the most likely causes of osteoporosis.

How to treat osteoporosis in men

Several drugs have been recently been approved for osteoporosis treatment in men. With regards to bisphosphonates, 10mg daily of alendronate or 35mg weekly of risedronate are the most frequently prescribed drug treatments. These drugs have been shown to exert inhibitory effects on osteoclasts, the cells in charge of bone resorption. In clinical trials, these drugs have proven to be effective in preventing bone fractures.

Testosterone therapy

Approximately 15% of men present secondary osteoporosis due to hypogonadism. Testosterone, the main male hormone, has been shown to stimulate bone and muscle growth. A testosterone deficiency is thus likely to have an impact on bone quality and lead to osteoporosis. If you are suffering from this condition, your doctor may prescribe testosterone therapy.

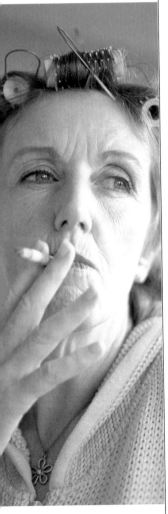

Risk factors for osteoporosis

Numerous factors have been shown to have an influence on bone mass. While some of these factors are out of our control, others are linked to our lifestyle and may be controlled. Osteoporosis often strikes in patients who display several risk factors at the same time.

General factors

Age is certainly a risk factor for osteoporosis. Although the disease is rare in younger individuals, the occurrence of osteoporosis has been shown to significantly and continuously increase after age 50. Furthermore, women are at greater risk than men, especially after menopause.

Genetic factors also play a role, as children of parents suffering from osteoporosis present a lower bone mineral density and are thus more likely to develop the disease themselves.

The risk of osteoporosis is increased in individuals of small size and low body weight, and in those presenting endocrine disorders such as hyperthyroidism or Cushing's syndrome, inflammatory disorders such as rheumatoid arthritis or ankylosing spondylarthritis, or gastrointestinal disorders, including liver disease.

Habits you can change

Osteoporosis is often associated with a poor diet: an insufficient consumption of milk and dairy products may lead to calcium deficiency, which is likely to damage bones. Excessive alcohol consumption slows down new bone growth and the production of sex hormones, and excessive consumption of salt, caffeine, or protein favors the excretion of calcium in the urine.

Additionally, smoking plays a major role in bone weakness and vulnerability to fracture. Moreover, in women, cigarette smoking may induce menopause at an earlier age. During menopause, the production of female hormones such as estrogen and progesterone begins to decline, and so estrogens are no longer able to protect bones against osteoporosis. Physical activity has also been shown to play a significant role in preventing osteoporosis. Thus, lack of exercise has negative effects on bones, though excessively strenuous physical activities may also make women vulnerable to osteoporosis.

Lack of exposure to the sun is widely considered to be the primary cause of vitamin D deficiency.

Vitamin D is produced in the skin in response to the sun's ultraviolet rays. Vitamin D is essential for promoting calcium absorption in the digestive tract and enhances its binding to the bones.

Certain drugs, such corticosteroids taken for a long time and at high dose levels provoke a decrease in bone mass, contributing to the occurrence of secondary osteoporosis and fragility fractures. These drugs are widely used to treat inflammatory conditions such as rheumatoid arthritis or skin eczema, or to prevent asthma attacks. Likewise, prolonged treatment with anticonvulsant drugs in the case of epilepsy has been shown to have negative effects on bone strength. If taken over prolonged periods, heparin, an anticoagulant used in the prevention and treatment of venous thrombosis, increases the risk of osteoporosis. Lastly, GnRH agonists, which are prescribed for the treatment of certain cancers or gynecological disorders, have also been associated with increased risk for osteoporosis.

WHO classification of BMI

WHO has established a classification with cut-off points to differentiate underweight, normal weight, overweight, and obesity:

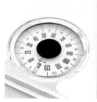

BMI	CLASSIFICATION
<18.5	Underweight
18.5 to 25	Normal
25 to 30	Overweight
30 to 35	Moderate obesity
35 to 40	Severe obesity
>40	Morbid obesity

What are the symptoms of osteoporosis?

The hallmark of osteoporosis, reduced bone mass, progresses silently. In the absence of resulting complications, it is not associated with any pain or other physical discomfort, contrary to popular belief.

Silent until complications occur

Osteoporosis is a silent disease, which means that the reduction in bone mass does not provoke any obvious symptoms. Therefore, numerous patients affected by osteoporosis are unaware of their condition until complications occur. Bone fractures are the most common complications: bones weakened by osteoporosis are easily broken, following a minor injury or even spontaneously. Although fractures may occur anywhere, the bones that are broken the most often are those of the hip, spine, and wrist.

The most common fractures

Wrist fractures, an early complication of osteoporosis, often occur between the ages of 50 and 60 years, and should be seen as a "warning sign" for osteoporosis. This type of fracture generally occurs when one catches him or herself in a fall with an outstretched hand. Vertebral fractures, also known as compression fractures, are characterized by a collapse of the central vertebral endplate due to pressure from the intervertebral discs. This usually happens in the middle and lower back, involving dorsal and lumbar vertebrae. Cervical vertebrae, which form the cervical spine at the base of the skull, are rarely involved.

Femoral head fractures, which are commonly referred to as hip fractures, are one of the most feared complications of osteoporosis, as they mainly affect the very elderly. Hip fracture requires immediate surgery. Nevertheless, full functional recovery is likely to occur in only 20% of all cases following surgery. Most patients experience permanent disability, and limping is one of the major complaints. These fractures mostly occur after a fall, but spontaneous fractures may also be observed in severe osteoporosis.

When to test for osteoporosis?

As osteoporosis is a silent disease, it is often not diagnosed until fractures occur. Osteoporosis should be suspected in case of repeated fractures, fractures occurring after age 50, or fractures following a fall or other injury. A decrease in height of more than 3cm, and the presence of significant pain or deformation of the spine are all warning signs of osteoporosis.

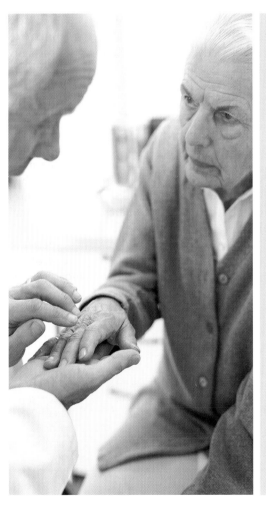

When a decrease in height and Dowager's hump are involved

Vertebral fractures may produce symptoms in addition to pain, such as a decrease in height, which may progress over several years. As the spinal bones weaken, they often collapse, leading to loss of height and a stooped posture, also known as "Dowager's hump". This deformity, which is often mistaken for normal aging, may in turn cause other problems, such as respiratory difficulties, acid reflux disease, or a sensation of permanent abdominal constriction and pain. Apart from these physical signs, vertebral fractures may also have significant psychological effects and may lead to loss of self-esteem. The quality of life of patients suffering from vertebral fractures has been shown to be significantly poorer. With the passage of time, patients become physically unable to adequately take care of look themselves and must be admitted to nursing homes.

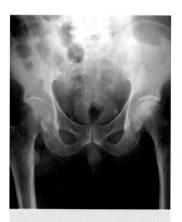

Risk factors for fractures

Factors that increase the likelihood of developing broken bones are called risk factors. To date, numerous risk factors for osteoporosis have been identified. The best method of detecting osteoporosis is to have a bone mineral density test. This test measures bone density at multiple sites of the body. Clinical studies have clearly shown that the risk of suffering from bone fractures, along with their serious effects on mobility and quality of life, increases when bone mineral density decreases.

Osteoporosis: facts and figures

Osteoporosis worldwide:
• After age 50, one out of every three women and one out of every five men suffer from osteoporosis.
• Approximately 1.6 million hip fractures occur every year.
• It is predicted that the number of fractures due to osteoporosis will increase to more than 3 million by 2025.
• Only one out of three elderly patients regains the level of independence he or she had prior to the injury.

Reference: International Osteoporosis Foundation. Report 2007

Prior to prescribing any drug therapy, your doctor will probably examine not only your bone mineral density but also other risk factors. In other words, the decision to begin treatment depends not only on the results of your bone mineral density tests but also on other risk factors. For example, if you have been receiving corticosteroids for a long time, your doctor may give you a preventive prescription of a bisphosphonate drug, even if your T-score is above or equal to -1.5. In contrast, if you have already experienced a bone fracture, your doctor will probably prescribe medication, regardless of your T-score value.

Factors related to bone mineral density

Estrogen deficiency during menopause is considered a major risk factor for osteoporosis, especially if menopause occurs before age 40.

Other risk factors potentially leading to osteoporosis are: slim patients with a body mass index <19 kg/m², family history of hip fractures, history of minor injuries, and prolonged periods of immobilization. Elderly patients and those having undergone prolonged corticosteroid treatment are also more prone to osteoporotic fractures. Lastly, insufficient dietary intake of calcium and vitamin D, along with reduced sun exposure, may increase your risk of developing osteoporotic fractures, especially later in life.

Factors related to bone mineral density

- Estrogen deficiency
- Low body mass index (<19kg/m²)
- Caucasian race
- Advanced age
- Low calcium intake in diet

- Family history of hip fractures
- Past history of minor injuries
- Prolonged corticosteroid treatment
- Prolonged immobilization
- Radiological signs of osteopenia

Factors unrelated to bone mineral density

Balance and coordination disorders as well as vision problems are included in this category. A reduction in lean body mass and a sedentary lifestyle are also risk factors, as is the use of tranquilizers and other psychotropic drugs, which may cause elderly patients to lose their balance and fall.

Factors unrelated to bone mineral density

- Balance and coordination disorders
- Vision problems
- Reduction in lean body mass

- Sedentary lifestyle
- Use of tranquilizers
- Cerebrovascular problems

Hip fracture

Proximal femoral fractures, also known as hip fractures, are very common in elderly patients. They are rare in patients under the age 70, and their frequency then increases exponentially with age. Over recent decades, the frequency of hip fractures has increased dramatically, and their occurrence is expected to continue to rise in future years, due to an ageing population.

What is a hip fracture?

The thigh extends from the hip to the knee, and its bone is the called the femur. At the knee joint, the femur joins the tibia and kneecap, which lies in front of the knee joint. At its upper end, the femur joins hip bone to form the hip joint. It is precisely at this upper end of the femur, which becomes very delicate and fragile as its density decreases with age, that the risk of fracture is the highest.

What are the symptoms of a hip fracture?

It is hard to miss the symptoms of a hip fracture as, they are rather obvious. First, the patient has recently fallen. This is followed by a sudden hip pain, associated with the inability to elevate the leg or walk. However, sometimes stress fractures also occur in the absence of major trauma. Patients with hip stress fractures often complain of persistent pain in the hip, which intensifies when weight is placed on that leg.

How is osteoporosis diagnosed?

During diagnosis, your doctor will begin by asking you questions about your medical history and your

Hip fractures: facts and figures

In the United States, more than 350 000 hip fractures are reported every year, and this number is expected to triple by 2050. A recent publication reported that 81% of patients with hip fractures were older than 75 years, and 43% older than 85. These hip fractures are associated with high morbidity and mortality rates, as 15-20% of patients die within 1 year of their fracture and more than half do not regain the activity level they had prior to their injury.

Hip joint

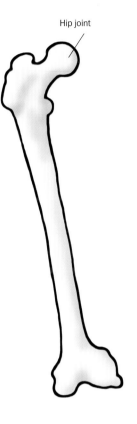

current symptoms. He or she will then perform a physical examination to try and find a link between your symptoms and physical findings. This will be followed by a X-ray of your hip, which will be performed by a qualified radiology technician. These images will allow the reader to recognize the type of fracture and its exact location. In some cases, conventional X-rays do not suffice in providing diagnostic information, and bone scintigraphy or magnetic resonance imaging (MRI) may be required.

As far as treatment is concerned, immediate surgery is the first course of action, as it both relieves pain and helps preserve the patient's mobility. However, some patients are unable to tolerate anesthesia for such a procedure due to medical problems, such as a recent heart attack. Should this be the case, the surgery may be postponed. Functional recovery after hip fracture is often poorer in men than women.

Bone scintigraphy

To perform a bone scintigraphy, the nuclear medicine specialist intravenously injects very small amounts of a radioactive element into your bloodstream. This radioactive element is then absorbed by your skeleton, and the nuclear medicine specialist uses a gamma-camera to trace its distribution throughout your body.

Bone scintigraphy is a painless procedure that tests for fractures. In the case of a fracture, there will be an increased focal uptake of the radiotracer at the site of the fracture, enabling your physician to make a correct diagnosis.

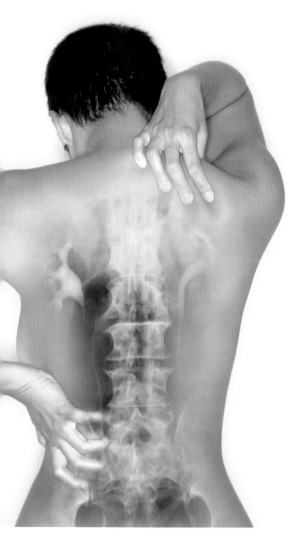

Other common fractures

In addition to hip fractures, osteoporotic fractures may also involve other bones such as the vertebrae or the wrist.

Compression fractures of the spine

Unlike stress fractures, compression fractures are complete fractures that disrupt the bone tissue, resulting in the collapse of the affected bone. The most common site of compression fractures is in the vertebrae, particularly at the thoracic and lumbar spine level. Most fractures are associated with intense pain, particularly in the sitting or standing position. If compression fractures occur over time at several levels of the spine, they reduce the height of the spine. In this case, the person becomes shorter and presents a typical deformation of the spine, with an outward curvature known as cyphosis or Dowager's hump. This spinal deformation may cause significant pain and disabilities in everyday-life situations, as well as breathing, balance, and mobility problems.

While most fractures are associated with intense pain, others go unnoticed, especially in the very elderly. Therefore, radiological signs of compression fractures may be detected in patients who have had no pain or other symptoms, and with no history of a fall or traumatic event. Yet, it has been shown in clinical studies that vertebral fractures, even if they are asymptomatic and go unnoticed, have a negative impact on the patient's quality of life.

Initially, bed rest may be indicated to relieve pain. Physiotherapy may be very useful as it allows the patient to strengthen his or her muscles, and by doing so, help preserve mobility. In the same context, patients should be encouraged to get up and walk as soon as possible. Wearing a brace does not prevent spinal deformation but may be effective for relieving pain.

Wrist fractures

The wrist is made up of two bones, the radius and the ulna. The most common form of wrist fracture causes the radius to break and bend away from the palm. If this happens, the patient may notice a change in the shape of his or her wrist. This fracture is also known as Colles's fracture or Putteau's fracture, after the two surgeons who first described this condition. The usual cause of such a fracture is a fall, in which the person falling tries to break his or her fall with his or her hands, and the wrist is forced backwards. In nine out of ten postmenopausal women presenting wrist fractures, osteoporosis is the underlying cause. This type of fracture may be isolated or associated with other, even more disabling fractures, such as those of the hip or vertebrae. Should this be the case, the likelihood of osteoporosis being the primary cause is even higher. Thus, if you are postmenopausal and suffer from a wrist fracture, it is crucial that you undergo a bone density test, so that your doctor can confirm or rule out osteoporosis. Common symptoms of a wrist fracture include immediate swelling and localized pain, which is at times associated with a crackling sound or sensation. Upon examination, the wrist presents the classic "dinner fork" appearance. X-rays allow the doctor to confirm this diagnosis by revealing the backward movement of the lower end of the radius.

Management of wrist fractures

Treatment for wrist fractures consists of repositioning of the bone. To this end, the bone fragments are repositioned into their correct anatomic position and held together by a plaster cast until they fuse back together. During recovery, regular x-rays must be performed in order to monitor the fracture and ensure that no dislocation has occurred. In some cases, surgical treatment may be considered. Different surgical options are available, including a reduction of the fracture followed by either internal fixation using a reconstruction plate and screws, or by external fixation with pins placed in the bone fragments.

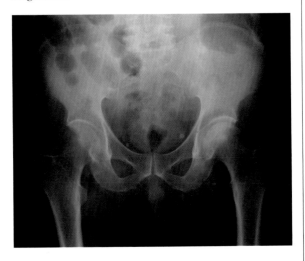

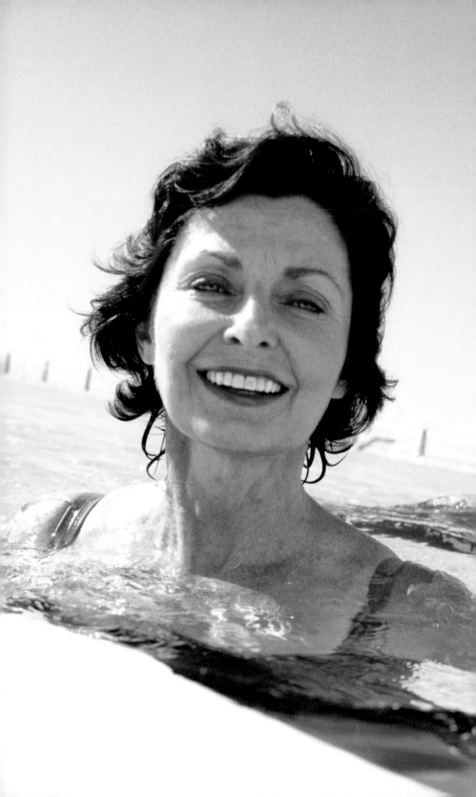

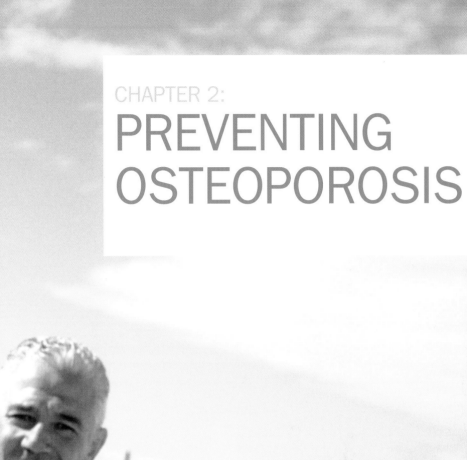

CHAPTER 2

PREVENTING OSTEOPOROSIS

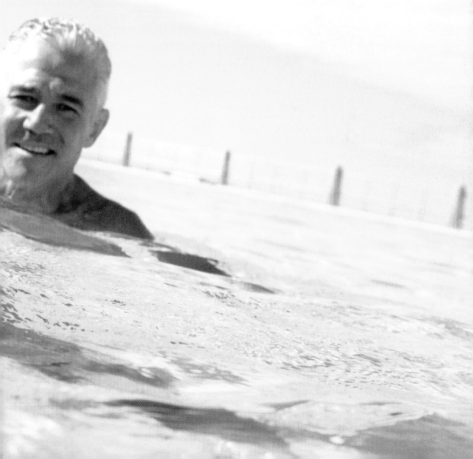

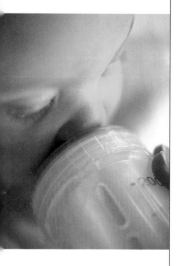

PREVENTING OSTEOPOROSIS

Prevention for each age group

Bone mass builds up progressively during childhood and adolescence, reaching a peak at around 20 years, which is also referred to as maximum bone mass. For approximately 10 years, bone mass stabilizes at this plateau. From age 30 and beyond, bone mass begins to decline at a rate depending on individual patients and conditions.

Childhood and adolescence

During this period, regular physical exercise is highly recommended, as it strengthens bones. It is important to build up bone mass early in life in order to decrease the child's risk of developing osteoporosis later in life. The more earlier exercise begins, the better, as maximum bone mass will be greater. Calcium, vitamin D, and proteins are essential nutrients that your body needs on a daily basis to strengthen bones. Children need plenty of calcium! The best source of calcium is low-fat dairy products such as low-fat yogurt and cheese. Smaller amounts of calcium are also found in broccoli, green and leafy vegetables, and kidney beans. Sun exposure is also important: the vitamin D produced by sunlight under your skin is essential for your bone density. It is important to eat a balanced diet and avoid salty foods such as ready-

Get regular exercise

Lack of physical exercise is a well-known risk factor for osteoporosis. Physical exercise improves bone mineral density and is beneficial at any age. It is recommended that you regularly engage in activities such as walking or jogging. Try to vary your activities in order to place your bones under different types of mechanical strain.

made dishes or food containing excessive animal proteins (meat, fish, and eggs) which make the body excrete calcium through the urine.

Adulthood

In addition to consuming plenty of low-fat dairy products and getting regular exercise, avoid smoking and consume alcohol in moderation (no more than two drinks per day), if at all, in order to reduce your risk for osteoporosis. Nicotine is toxic for your body, as it stimulates your sympathetic nervous system and can cause inflammatory diseases. Alcohol may damage the cells responsible for building and repairing bone tissue.

Menopause

A diet that is too high in acids may aggravate the loss of bone tissue. In order to avoid the acidification of your body, make sure that you do not eat too much grain, red meat, fish, or cheese, and that you eat plenty of fruits and vegetables. It is recommended that you take at least 1000mg of calcium per day. Of course, you must not forget to get enough regular physical exercise. Avoid tobacco and consume alcohol only in moderation, if at all.

Old age

In the elderly, preventive measures include a balanced diet and physical exercise. After age 65, daily calcium intake should reach 1200mg. In practice, the consumption of dairy products, fruit, grains, and mineral water rich in calcium can meet daily requirements. If you are unable to fulfill this, a calcium supplement may be prescribed by your physician.

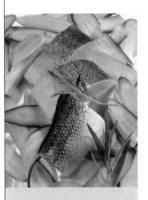

With no sun, no vitamin D

Vitamin D is found in food such as oily fish, cheese, and egg yolks, but it is largely produced by the skin. When exposed to ultraviolet rays, the skin creates vitamin D, which increases calcium absorption by the intestines, and its binding to the bones.

The role of food

A healthy diet plays a significant role in the prevention and treatment of osteoporosis. Thus, it is important to understand what a healthy diet is, and how you can make good choices.

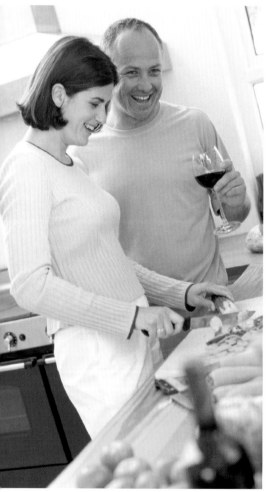

A healthy and balanced diet

First of all, let us take a look at what a balanced diet is. A balanced diet should provide your body with all of its needs in terms of carbohydrates, fats, and proteins, as well as vitamins, minerals, and trace elements. Today, our diet is heavy in red meat, fish, and grain. Even if these meats contain the animal proteins that your body needs, they also have a high fat content, particularly the saturated fats responsible for bad cholesterol and cardiovascular diseases. Fish, on the other hand, contain unsaturated fats, which may be very beneficial for the body.

Maintaining a healthy and balanced diet does not only mean limiting fat intake. This also means consuming plenty of vitamins and minerals, as well as essential fibers. In addition to their high potassium levels, fruits and vegetables are also rich in antioxidants such as vitamins C and E, minerals like calcium and magnesium, as well as fibers, which promote digestion. Watch your diet carefully, but this does not mean that you need to stop eating meat entirely. Moderation is the key. Eat more fish and white meat, and less red meat. Make sure to include fruit and vegetables at every meal.

Avoid strict diets

Being vegetarian means eating only plant products, and in some cases animal products such as dairy, eggs, or fish. A vegan diet excludes all animal products and does not permit the consumption of dairy, meat, eggs, or fish. This diet can be very dangerous, as it deprives your body of essential amino acids and vitamin D, which are contained in fish and meat. It also deprives you of calcium, which is necessary for your bones. In the long term, a vegan diet can lead to osteoporosis. Fruits, vegetables, and grains do contain amino acids, but they cannot meet all your needs alone. In conclusion, the most important thing to keep in mind is balance and moderation.

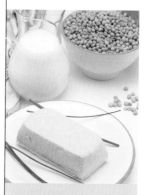

The role of proteins

Proteins play an essential role in preventing osteoporosis. They help bind calcium to the bones, and slow the aging of cells. Proteins are made up of amino acids linked together according to their number and order, which determine the protein's role. For a balanced diet, it is important to consume both animal proteins such as fish and meat, and vegetable proteins, from soy, legumes, and grains.

Drink enough milk

Milk is an excellent source of calcium. One liter of cow's milk contains about 1000mg of calcium. This mineral is essential for your general health, and especially for your bones. It is instrumental in preventing osteoporosis. Our bones are comprised of collagen fibers which are solidified thanks to calcium salts. When you do not consume enough calcium, your body must take calcium from your bone tissue reserves in order to maintain stable levels of calcium in your blood. In contrast to many cheeses, milk has the advantage of not having been transformed into acids during digestion.

Diet and bones' health

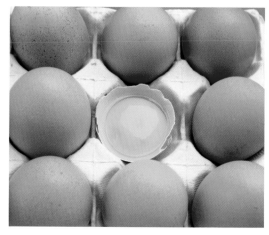

A balanced diet with an adequate intake of calcium, vitamin D and proteins, contributes to maintaining healthy bones and preventing osteoporosis.

Calcium's key role

Bone formation depends on calcium. Make sure you are getting enough calcium so that your body does not need to use up its reserves- mainly from the bones- in order to maintain a stable level of calcium in the blood. There are many dietary sources of calcium, especially milk and cheese, but also eggs, vegetables, fish, and certain mineral waters.

In children and adolescents, an appropriate calcium intake allows the body to increase peak bone mass, which has a lifelong impact on bone mineral density. Depending on the child or adolescent's age, the recommended daily allowance ranges from 800 to 1500mg. Adults, especially menopausal women and the elderly, need between 1200 and 1500mg per day in order counteract the negative effects of decreased estrogen levels.

Vitamin D, calcium's ally

Vitamin D is not a vitamin in the strictest sense of the term, as only 10% of the body's needs are covered by diet. Foods rich in vitamin D include egg yolks, oily fish, cheese, and butter. The other 90% is produced under the skin when it is exposed to sunlight. This is why it is important to be exposed to the sunlight for a minimum of 15 minutes every day.

Under the effect of vitamin D, calcium is absorbed in the body more rapidly, and it binds more effectively to the bones. The elderly are often very sedentary, and are those most affected by a vitamin D deficiency, which is often associated with a lack of calcium. In this case, a vitamin D and calcium supplement is often necessary.

Remember to eat your vegetables!

Contrary to common belief, fruits and vegetables also contain calcium, even if it is less than in dairy products. Moreover, fruits and vegetables also contain fibers, which have a beneficial effect on digestion. Many fruits and vegetables are also alkaline based, which means that they help preserve the acid-base balance in your body. Some even contain substances which mimic the effects of estrogens, and are known as phytoestrogens. These substances are beneficial for your bones. The main sources of phytoestrogens are legumes, particularly soy, and seaweed. The antioxidants present in fruits and vegetables, such as polyphenols, also play an important role. They decrease inflammation in the bones, and thereby fight osteoporosis.

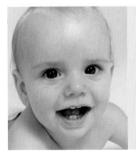

Vitamin D deficiency

A deficiency in vitamin D may lead to bone diseases. In children, a deficiency of vitamin D can lead to rickets, which is a condition in which mineral salts insufficiently bind to the bone. This condition has become rare in industrialized countries, as all newborn babies systematically receive vitamin D supplements. In adults, a vitamin D deficiency is a well-known risk factor for osteoporosis.

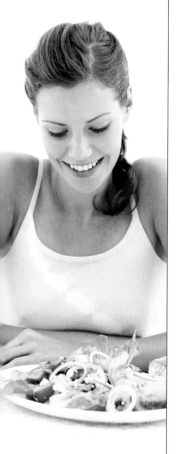

Other vitamins and minerals

Vitamins and minerals are found in many of the foods we eat, and allow us to remain in good health. The more varied our diet is, the more likely it is that we will fulfill the daily recommended allowance of vitamins and minerals.

Don't forget about minerals

Sodium and potassium are two essential minerals. Today, we tend to consume too much sodium and not enough potassium. Indeed, our modern diet contains much more salt, which is already present in food, whether we add it or not, such as in cold cuts, canned foods, chips, cheese, etc. Excess sodium does not only lead to hypertension, but it is also associated with the acidification of our tissues and our bodies. To ensure a better balance between sodium and potassium, decrease your consumption of salt and eat more fruits and vegetables, which are an excellent source of potassium.

Silica and magnesium are also essential for the prevention and treatment of osteoporosis. Studies have revealed a link between the insufficient consumption of silica, and certain diseases that affect connective tissue, including bones and tendons. Whole grain, fruit, and seafood contain low levels of silica. The main source of this mineral is mineral water, which is a good reason to drink at least 1.5 liters per day. In addition to its benefits for the nervous system, magnesium plays an important role in bone health. Today, magnesium deficiency is becoming an increasingly common problem, and can reduce bone mineral density. Sources of magnesium are not hard to find, and include whole grain, legumes, nuts, cacao, and mineral water.

Discover the benefits of vitamins

Vitamin D is essential for the bones as it promotes calcium absorption by the digestive tract and its binding to the bones. Only 10% of our recommended daily allowance of vitamin D is covered by our diet, for example with oily fish, cheese, and egg yolk. The remaining 90% is produced under the skin, under the effect of sunlight.

Vitamin B12 is responsible for the multiplication of cells, including osteoblasts, which are necessary for bone regeneration. A vitamin B12 deficiency in the blood can lead to lower bone mineral density. This vitamin is present in meat, offal, seafood, oily fish, and egg yolk.

Antioxidants such as vitamin C, which is mainly present in fruits and vegetables, are also instrumental in preventing osteoporosis. Vitamin C is essential as it allows for collagen to be synthesized. Collagen is a substance found in the bones. Vitamin B6 is also beneficial, as it contributes to the assimilation of magnesium by the tissues.

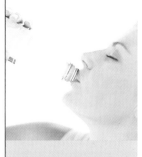

Drink plenty of mineral water

Drink mineral water instead of tap water, as this can be a good solution for those who do not consume many dairy products. You must choose a mineral water that is rich in calcium, as content varies from one brand to the next. Some mineral waters contain more than 500mg of calcium per liter. If you drink 1 to 1.5 liters per day, you would already be meeting a large part of the recommended daily allowance for calcium.

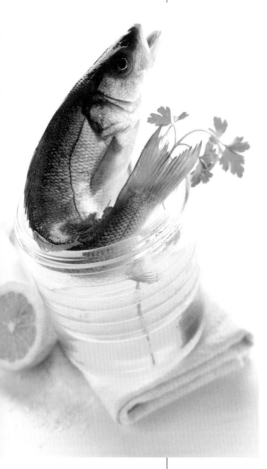

Which fats are good fats ?

We need to consume sufficient amounts of good fats, as they are necessary in order for our body to perform its vital functions. The problem, however, is excess fat! Knowing how to distinguish good fats from bad fats will allow you to choose a healthy and balanced diet.

What is the role that dietary fat plays?

Dietary fats, whether of animal or vegetable origin, are present in food items in the form of triglycerides. Each triglyceride molecule is made up of glycerol– an alcohol– and three fatty acids. While the glycerol portion makes up the backbone of the molecules, the fatty acids branch out from the glycerol portion. A fatty acid chain is made up of 12 to 22 carbon atoms. While saturated fatty acids have no carbon-carbon double bonds in their molecule, unsaturated fatty acids do have carbon-carbon double bonds in their molecule, and can incorporate additional hydrogen atoms.

Saturated fatty acids

Without any double bond, saturated fatty acids present a relatively rigid structure and are solid at room temperature. They are found in butter, whole milk, and cheese, but also as " hidden fat" in sausage, chips, cookies, and cake. Mainly found in animal products, these fatty acids are harmful to your health, as they have been shown to raise the cholesterol levels in the blood.

Excessive cholesterol in the blood leaves deposits on the artery wall, resulting in the formation of atherosclerotic plaque, and subsequently of athe-rosclerosis and coronary heart disease. We hope that now you understand better why it is important to limit your dietary intake of saturated fatty acids and cholesterol.

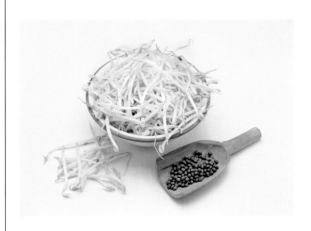

Unsaturated fatty acids

These fatty acids have at least one double bond between carbon atoms, and can thus incorporate additional hydrogen molecules. Depending on the number of carbon double bonds, unsaturated fatty acids are classified into monounsaturated fatty acids or omega-9 (one single double bond) and polyunsaturated fatty acids (several double bonds). Olive oil and hazelnut oil are very rich in omega 9. There are two major families of polyunsaturated fats: omega-3 and omega-6 fatty acids.

Fresh oily fish is one of the best and most convenient sources of omega-3 fatty acids, and includes salmon, halibut, tuna, and scallops. Other types of food that are omega 3 boosters are rapeseed oil, winter squash, walnuts, and soybeans. These omega-3 fatty acids are instrumental in protecting you against atherosclerosis. Therefore, keep focused on bringing more omega-3 rich food into your diet. In the modern diet, there are many sources of omega-6 fatty acids, essentially sunflower oil – the richest natural source-, corn oil, rapeseed oil, and soy oil. Animal omega-3 sources include lean meats, offal, and breast milk.

This class of polyunsaturated fatty acids has been shown to contribute to the production of inflammatory mediators, such as cytokines, and potentially accelerate the formation of atherosclerotic plaque in arterial walls.

These cytokines have also been associated with bone mineral loss, or in other words, osteoporosis. Therefore, if you wish to preserve your bone mass, you should preferably consume foods rich in omega-3 rather than omega-6 fatty acids.

Omega-3 fatty acids help prevent osteoporosis

Two fatty acids belonging to the omega-3 class play a major role in osteoporosis prevention: eicosapentaenoic acid (EPA) and docosahexaenoic acid (DHA). EPA and DHA are found in all oily fish and fish oils. Experiments showed that these acids limit the formation of cytokines, which play a role in inflammatory processes.

Dairy products: good or bad?

Milk is a whole food, used for producing other products: cheese, yogurt, butter, cream, etc. As milk is the main source of calcium, it is essential for the development and maintenance of our bones. Although dairy products are an important source of calcium, they are not all the same and some should even be avoided.

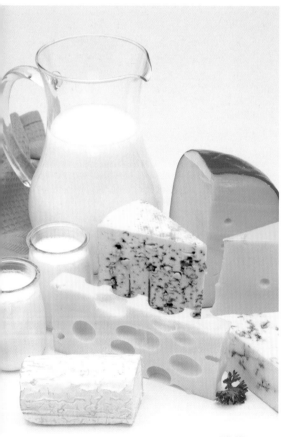

What does milk contain?

Milk is an excellent source of minerals such as calcium, phosphorus, potassium, and sodium. However, it lacks magnesium and iron. Milk contains the vitamins A, C, D, E, K, B1, B2, and PP. A number of these vitamins, specifically the fat-soluble vitamins A, D, E, and K, are not found in skim milk.
Milk contains numerous proteins and can therefore replace or complement meat and eggs. However, these proteins may cause allergies, especially in young children. They are also difficult to digest when combined with coffee, acidic foods, or fruit.

Butter, yogurt, cheese... the choice is endless

In its unprocessed form, yogurt has considerable benefits. Choose plain rather than flavored yogurt, which may be high in sugar. In order to decrease your risk of cardiovascular diseases, consume yogurt made from skim milk. Although cottage cheese has fewer benefits than yogurt, it has a remarkably high protein content, higher than that of yogurt.

When consumed in small quantities, cheese has a beneficial effect, because it is rich in calcium. Above all, consume cheese made from unpasteurized milk. Nevertheless, be careful of the fats found in cheese, especially if you are overweight or suffer from cardiovascular disease!

Apart from its vitamin content, butter is not very beneficial. It contains saturated fats and low levels of proteins and calcium. Therefore, do not overindulge in butter, or even better, avoid it.

Should we remove cheese from our plates?

No. Cheese is an excellent source of calcium and is therefore recommended, provided that it is consumed in moderation. You must also take into account that not all cheeses have the same nutritional value. Preferably, choose cooked cheese. These varieties of cheese are high in calcium, low in lactose, and therefore easy to digest. Pressed cheese, such as feta, unripened cheese, and cheese spreads, is also a good source of calcium. In short, although cheese is not off-limits, it is wise to limit your consumption. Certain experts recommend consuming a maximum of 50g daily. Try these tricks : cut cheese into small slices, spread it thinly, and use less cheese when you cook.

Which dairy products could be beneficial for osteoporosis sufferers?

Above all, avoid fatty and salty cheeses. This also applies to dairy desserts, which are often high in fat and sugar. It is better to choose plain yogurt made from skim or low-fat milk and low-fat cheese. If you love flavored yogurt, you can add fresh fruit to plain yogurt: this allows you to control the quality of the fruit as well as the amount of sugar you consume. If you are lactose intolerant, your doctor can prescribe a calcium supplement.

The truth about the acid-base balance

As we have become more sedentary and our dietary habits have changed, our body environment has progressively become acidic. While acidification is harmful to our bodies, there are steps we can take against it.

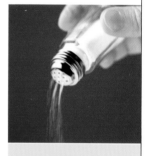

Salt in moderation

If salt is consumed in excessive amounts – more than 8.5g per day -, it is harmful to the body, because it depletes its calcium reserves. Through a hormonal process, calcium is added to the blood from calcium reserves in the bones. This surplus must then be excreted in the urine. Therefore, consume salt in moderation and, whenever possible, opt for unrefined grey salts.

Some definitions

Before we delve deeper into this topic, let us define pH. pH is a unit of measurement for the acidity or alkalinity of a body. It ranges from 0 to 14, 0 being the strongest level of acidity, 7 representing neutrality, and 14 being the highest level of alkalinity. When a solution has a pH lower than 7, it is considered "acidic". When a solution has a pH higher than 7, it is considered "alkaline" or "basic". In a healthy body, the blood's pH is slightly alkaline, approximately 7.4. Any variation in the pH is harmful to the body. Fortunately, the body has protective systems called "buffer systems", which allow it to maintain a constant pH level.

The foods we consume are either alkalizing or acidifying. It s important to note that acidity is not the same as a sour taste. Lemons may be sour to the taste, but they are only slightly acidifying because they release alkaline compounds into our bodies. Sugar is another example: white sugar is not at all acidic to the taste, but once it is digested, white sugar is transformed into acid.

Acidification is dangerous to our bodies

Our body's acidity is determined by the food we eat. Our modern Western diet is too acidifying. In order to remain healthy, our bodies must maintain the pH of its blood at 7.4. If we consume too many acids, the body must neutralize them with the help of buffer systems, so that the blood maintains its pH. The problem lies in the fact that our body takes these substances from our bones in the form of calcium citrate or calcium bicarbonate. Hence, the bones lose some of their calcium, becoming more fragile and vulnerable to osteoporosis.

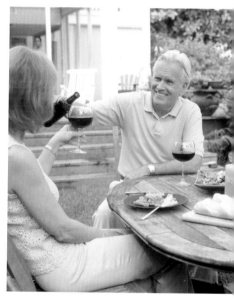

The mysteries of the acid-base balance

As we previously stated, acidification is harmful to the body. In order to keep your bones in good health, you should limit the causes of acidification. Maintaining an acid-base balance is an excellent way of doing this. This consists of watching your diet and choosing alkalinizing foods, especially fruit and vegetables. Do not overindulge in acidifying foods. Every time you consume a serving of an acidifying food, you should compensate for it with two servings of alkalizing foods: this is called the "two for one" rule. Keep in mind that in order to avoid acidifying your body, you should eat about 70% alkalinizing foods and about 30% acidifying foods.

How else does an acid-base imbalance affect the body?

Our body is designed in such a way that during the daytime, it stores the acids that it cannot excrete and then excretes them at night. When we take in excessive amounts of acids over a long period of time, certain substances (uric acid, urea, etc.) are not sufficiently excreted and accumulate in our body. With time, they irritate tissues, causing inflammation and damage, due to their toxic properties.

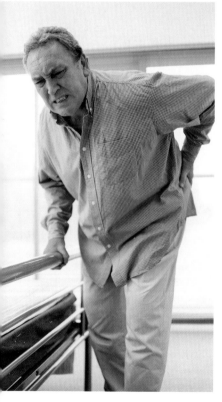

Rheumatoid diseases

Excess acid may cause the formation of crystals in the joints and can cause severe pain. The most striking example is gout, an inflammatory disease which mainly affects the joint in the big toe, but also that of the knees, feet, ankles, hands and elbows. The joint becomes red, hot, and swollen. Although treatment of gout calls for colchicine, a very effective drug, prevention is mostly based on dietary measures: cutting out foods that are acidic or acid-producing, limiting your consumption of fat, and a low-calorie diet if you are overweight.

An acidic environment may expose you to other rheumatoid diseases, such as arthritis and arthrosis, to give two examples. While arthritis is an inflammation of the joints, arthrosis is caused by a gradual degeneration of cartilage in the joints and by the deterioration of the bone directly underneath it. Apart from drug treatment using painkillers and anti-inflammatories, regaining an acid-base balance can be very useful. Correcting the acidic environment may help relieve chronic pain linked to rheumatoid diseases and may help slow down their progression.

Skin problems

Much like the kidneys and lungs, the skin is also a highly efficient organ which allows the body to excrete acids. The level of acids which have accumulated in the body therefore depends on the correct functioning of these tissues and organs. However, if the environment is very acidic, the acids excreted in sweat will eventually irritate the epidermis. The areas of the skin where a lot of sweating occurs are particularly vulnerable, because fissures and cracks may appear. According to certain experts, skin diseases such as eczema may be the result of an acidic environment. Moreover, dry skin may quite simply be a reflection of an acid-base imbalance. An excessively acidic environment also seems to expose the scalp to dandruff and itching. The acids excreted in sweat irritates the scalp, the latter becoming even drier. The skin flakes off more rapidly, and cells stick together, forming flakes which easily fall off.

Diet and tendinitis

Several nutritional factors contribute to tendon inflammation, or tendinitis. Acids, including uric acid, which is produced during the digestion of certain types of meat, are the main culprit. It was proven, that uric acid levels in people suffering from tendinitis were above normal levels. As diets which are too high in protein contribute to the acidification of the body environment, they could make you vulnerable to tendinitis. Moreover, contrary to muscles, tendons do not become enlarged if the protein intake is high. An imbalance between muscles and tendons may occur, which could be the cause of inflammation.

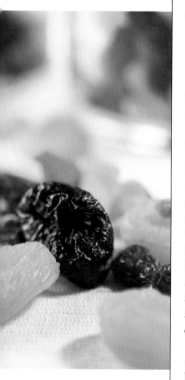

The acid-base balance in practice

In practice, a few simple steps allow us to recover our acid-base balance and therefore remain in good health.

How can I recover my acid-base balance?

• **Reduce your acid intake!** In order to do this you can limit your consumption of acidifying foods as much as possible, or even cut them out entirely for a short period of time – two weeks at most. Then, reintroduce them into your diet until you have found the right balance for your body. You can also limit the effect of acids on your body by following a simple rule: remember to always compensate a serving of acidifying food with two servings of alkalinizing foods. Take note of the fact that this diet is only efficient if it is followed long-term.

• **Eliminate the acids stored in your body!** The lungs are what one calls emunctories: they make it possible to excrete acids in the form of carbon dioxide. Physical exercise increases the heart rate and breathing and the more oxygen the lungs take in, the more acids can be excreted. To be most beneficial, physical exercise must be regular and sustained for a considerable amount of time.

• **Eat plenty of alkalinizing foods!** The bases found in alkalinizing foods help your body to rebuild itself. They act as acid buffers. This way, because your body no longer has to take from its bone reserves in order to excrete acids, you are protecting yourself from osteoporosis.

Alkalinizing and acidifying foods

The following are among the most acidifying foods: meat, fish, eggs, cheese, dairy products rich in fermented whey such as yogurt, vegetable oils, grains, legumes such as soy and white kidney beans, sugar, certain drinks such as coffee, tea, wine, and sodas.

Some sour-tasting foods also contribute to the body's acidification, for example, vegetables like tomatoes, rhubarb, acidic, unripe, or overripe fruit, honey and vinegar.

Alkalinizing foods contain only very few or no acids, and are rich in bases. These foods include potatoes, green and colorful vegetables – except for tomatoes –, cream, bananas, almonds, chestnuts, dried fruit, and bicarbonate-rich mineral water.

A few winning dietary steps

The ideal combination of foods are based on a balance between acids and bases. Ideally, you should consume 70% bases and 30% acids, that is, 2 bases for every acid, in order to follow what is called the "two-for-one" rule.

Combine cheese or grains with salad or fruit, and eat your steak with fresh vegetables or a soup. Replace the traditional meat sauce on your spaghetti with a vegetable sauce: this compensates for the pasta's acidity. Also, do not forget about the benefits of salads made up of raw vegetables – celery, beets, and carrots, for example – and potatoes, for their alkalinizing property, and a bit of cheese or an egg for their acidifying property.

Budwig cream for breakfast

Budwig cream is a healthy and energizing breakfast food. It consists of:
- 4 teaspoons of cottage cheese,
- 2 teaspoons of vegetable oil (flaxseed, wheat germ, sunflower, etc.);
- the juice of half a lemon;
- 1 banana;
- 1 seasonal fruit;
- 2 teaspoons of whole grain (oats, barley, wheat germ, etc.);
- 1 teaspoon of oily seeds (almonds, hazelnuts, or walnuts).

A day in the life of the acid-base balance regimen

Fruit and vegetables first

Apart from their alkalinizing properties, fruit and vegetables are excellent sources of antioxidants, which are very useful for the prevention of osteoporosis. The main antioxidants contained in fruit and vegetables are polyphenols and vitamins C and E. Polyphenols inhibit the damaging action that osteoclasts have on bones, and support the action of osteoblasts.

Different types of polyphenols help fight against osteoporosis: quercetin in apples, onions, and citrus fruit; anthocyanins and anthocyanosides in plums, bilberries, and dried prunes. Vitamin C is essential for bones and helps to build the collagen base which mineral salts bind to in order to form the bones. Vitamin C is found in citrus fruit, strawberries, and peppers. Vitamin E, which is found in almonds, hazelnuts, and wheat germ, protects cells and delays their aging.

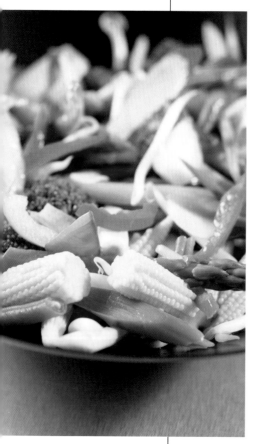

Breakfast suggestions

A balanced breakfast should include a hot drink, whole grain, butter or jam, a dairy product, and a serving of fruit. You can replace the fruit with a fresh fruit juice, but rather choose non-acidic seasonal fruit, such as pears, bananas, or apples.

Sweet breakfast: whole grain cereal, milk (soy or cow's milk), bread or whole-wheat toast, butter, tea.

Salty breakfast: an egg or portion of cooked ham, whole-wheat bread, cooked cheese, fruit.

Lunch suggestions

In order to make sure that you have a balanced intake of acids and bases, lunch should consist of raw vegetables (carrots, beets, celery, cabbage, etc.), animal protein (meat, fish, eggs), vegetables, starch (potatoes), and a fruit.

Lunch A : Raw endive and beetroot salad, steamed salmon, zucchini, stewed apples.

Lunch B : Tomato and radish salad, chicken breast with lemon and rosemary, spinach, a slice of whole-wheat bread, banana.

Lunch C : Tomato salad, hard-boiled egg, cucumber, and bean sprouts, a slice of whole-wheat bread, soft goat cheese, dried apricots.

Dinner suggestions

An ideal dinner should exclude animal proteins, as they are difficult to digest. It should consist of: a starter of vegetables; a main meal of vegetables with grains, eggs, or starch; and low-fat cheese, cottage cheese, or fruit.

Dinner A : hot vegetable soup, crushed potato and vegetable patty, and cottage cheese.

Dinner B : lentil salad, leek quiche, and fruit salad.

Dinner C : cold vegetable soup, gnocchi with cheese, and raspberries.

Remember to eat dinner relatively early, so that you have digested your meal before going to bed, allowing your kidneys to focus on detoxifying the body during the course of the night.

Nuts

Certain types of nuts, such as macadamia, Brazil nuts, or pecans, as well as hazelnuts, contain minerals - calcium, potassium, and magnesium -, trace elements – copper and zinc –, and vitamin E.

They are also sources of monounsaturated fatty acids which are beneficial for your health. It is therefore recommended to consume a handful of nuts every day.

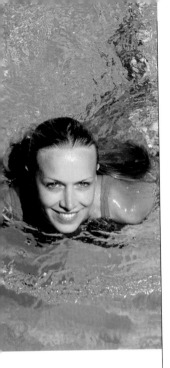

Exercise!

Physical exercise is vital for osteoporosis prevention, but be careful not to overdo it.

Strong bones

When you get physical exercise, there are two forces acting on your bones: compression and traction. When you walk, for example, your bones carry the weight of your body and are compressed. Running involves two forces. Traction acts on the joints when your muscles contract in order to move your limbs. By wanting to resist this force, bones become stronger and therefore less vulnerable to osteoporosis. You can increase the benefits of exercise for your bones if you engage in various physical activities.

As you age, you get less and less physical exercise and become more sedentary. Your bones are exposed to only weak forces, or none at all, and bone tissue decreases and becomes fragile. While bone loss is an inevitable phenomenon linked to age, it is vital that you do not to worsen the situation. In order to maintain good bone health, get regular exercise.

Which sports carry the greatest benefits ?

"High-impact" activities, where your skeleton must carry all your body weight, are the most beneficial. Walking or running are good examples of this. However, not all "high-impact" activities have

Activities to avoid

You should avoid activities which could easily cause you to fall, and consequently, fracture a bone. Skiing, for example, is strongly discouraged. If you like cycling, avoid muddy and uneven ground. Activities which involve carrying heavy objects should also be avoided as they can lead to spinal compression fractures.

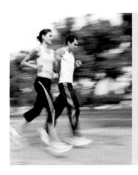

Get some fresh air!

Oxygenation contributes to the de-acidification of our bodies. When you engage in physical activity, your heart rate and need for oxygen increase. As the air outside is richer in oxygen than the air inside, your lungs take in more oxygen and can excrete more acids in the form of carbon dioxide.

the same effect on the skeleton. Speedwalking carries greater benefits than a simple leisurely stroll because your bones need to put up greater resistance. "Low-impact" activities can also prove useful, as is the case of weight training. Swimming is particularly encouraged if you suffer from pain due to bone fractures.

Most importantly, you should strengthen the bones which have been the most affected by osteoporosis: the wrists, spine, and hip. In order to do this, you can work your forearms, hips, back, and thighs. The sessions do not have to be very long, but in order to be beneficial, these exercises must be performed regularly. Adding weights during these exercises may increase the benefits for your skeleton.

Do not overdo it

Although physical exercise helps to prevent osteoporosis, be careful not to overdo it. In adolescents, dancers and gymnasts, for example, overexercising may lead to menstrual problems – amenorrhea –, often aggravated by restrictive weight-loss diets. Overexercising can also have harmful effects on joints. It is recommended not to lift heavy weights, so as to protect the spine.

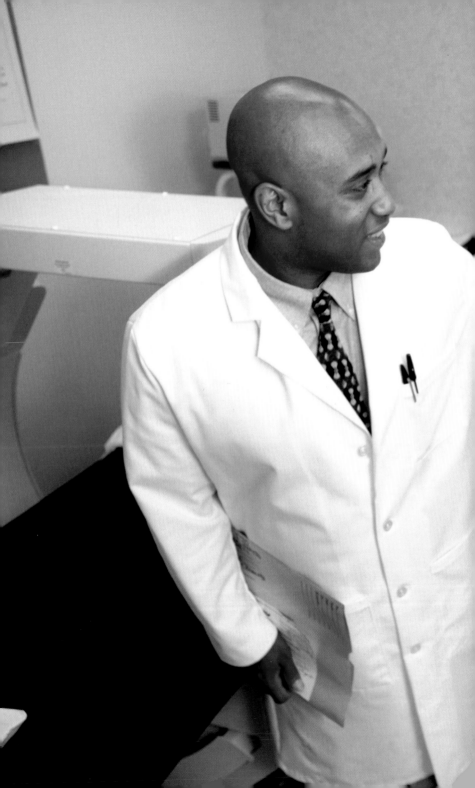

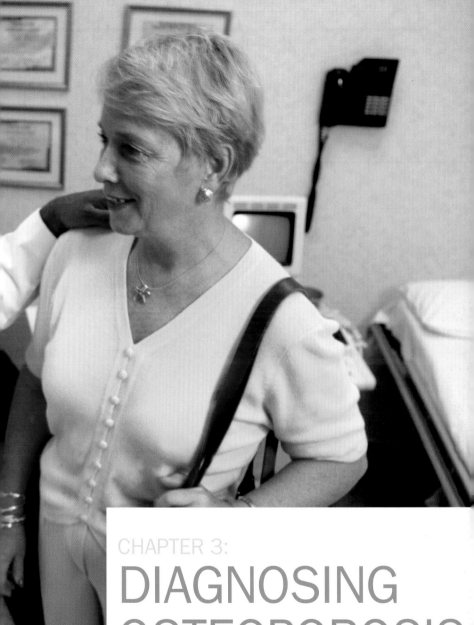

CHAPTER 3:

DIAGNOSING OSTEOPOROSIS

DIAGNOSING OSTEOPOROSIS

Screening

Osteoporosis is a very common disease. It is important to know when to get screened. In fact, screening often prevents the disease from worsening, and allows you to avoid extremely painful osteoporotic fractures.

Who should get screened?

Osteoporosis is essentially a disease affecting women of menopausal age. Screening therefore concerns, above all, women. While systematic screening for all menopausal women is hardly possible from a practical point of view, this

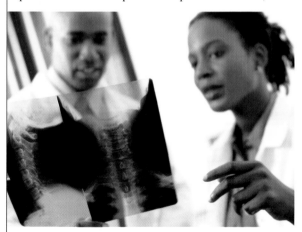

screening may be advised if there are additional risk factors. A wrist fracture in a menopausal woman is a clear indication that her bone mineral density should be measured.

However, screening does not exclusively affect menopausal women, because other people, such as individuals whose parents have fractured their femoral head or suffered spinal compression fractures which did not result from a strong impact. As family history plays a predominant role in osteoporosis, these individuals are more at risk of suffering an osteoporotic fracture.

Lastly, if you suffer from a disease causing you to need prolonged corticoid treatment– rheumatoid polyarthritis, asthma, multiple sclerosis, etc. –, screening is also necessary. Cortisone, the most well-known corticoid, lowers the absorption of calcium from food, and increases bone resorption, therefore increasing the risk of osteoporosis.

Which tests are used?

The principal diagnostic tool for osteoporosis is the bone densitometry test or bone mineral density test, using X-rays. Other medical imagining techniques are less useful in screening, though conventional X-rays are used to detect osteoporotic fractures.

Small spinal compression fractures, especially if they are linked to a size reduction of less than 20%, are difficult to detect on X-rays. CT (computed tomography) scanners or exams prove useful in this case. An MRI (magnetic resonance imaging) exam is performed when more time has passed following the spinal compression fracture. Laboratory analyses – of the blood and urine – may be very useful if osteoporosis has been diagnosed.

This allows physicians to rule out other bone diseases and secondary osteoporosis, and monitor the disease's progress.

What about screening programs?

The United States Preventive Services Task Force recommends that all women over 65 be screened regularly for osteoporosis, and that women who present risk factors such as being overweight or receiving hormone replacement therapy begin screening at age 60.

Nevertheless, every year in October, World Osteoporosis Day is held in approximately thirty countries. World Osteoporosis Day is an opportunity to increase awareness about this disease and advocate for better osteoporosis-related policies from governments and healthcare systems. In 2009 the slogan of World Osteoporosis Day was "Stand Tall for Bone Health!" Many employers in the United States regularly carry out osteoporosis screening and education programs in partnership with pharmaceutical companies.

Nutrition as a central theme in government action

The United States Department of Health and Human Services recognizes the importance of diet in preventing and treating osteoporosis. In August of 2009, the Institute of Medicine carried out a study on calcium, aimed at updating the 1989 Recommended Daily Allowances, thereby setting new standards for calcium intake in children ages 9 to 18.

Diagnosis

Your doctor may diagnose osteoporosis if certain risk factors are present: corticoid treatment, early menopause, thyroid alterations, etc. Sometimes osteoporosis is revealed by fractures caused by an impact, which may even be light. Nevertheless, bone mineral densitometry alone makes it possible to confirm the diagnosis of osteoporosis.

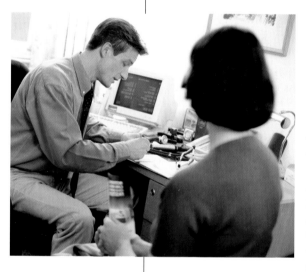

History-taking

Your doctor begins by asking you a series of questions which will allow him or her to detect possible risk factors. He or she will inquire about your dietary habits – anorexia nervosa, calcium and vitamin D deficiency – and about your lifestyle – whether you consume tobacco and alcohol on a regular basis and whether you have a sedentary lifestyle. Your doctor also examines your family history for fractures, especially those of the hip, or for osteoporosis in general. Because sex hormones play a major role in osteoporosis, your doctor will ask you about menopause and might also ask you about any long-term corticoid treatments that you may have undergone, as they are a recognized risk factor for osteoporosis. During the history-taking, your doctor will observe for any physical signs of osteoporosis: a considerable loss in spine size, or curvature of the spine.

Bone mineral density test

The bone mineral density test is a reference test for measuring bone mineral density, that is, the mineral content of bones. The test is usually performed on the spine, the femur, and sometimes also the wrist. The procedure is simple: you lie down on a table and your legs are positioned according to the purpose of the test. For example, if your spine is being tested, your legs will be raised using a cushion. The machine emits a beam of X-rays which passes through your bones and measures the amount of rays they absorb. The bone mineral density test provides precious information about bone density and bone mineral content. The denser the bone is, the more rays it absorbs. Take note of the fact that the machine emits a low-intensity beam and that the test is therefore not dangerous.

X-ray

X-rays make osteoporotic fractures, as well as major spinal compression fractures, visible. While the bone mineral density test is frequently performed for diagnosing a loss of bone mass, the X-ray technique is used to complete the results of the bone mineral density test. This test is particularly recommended in the case of a major reduction in spine size, an inwards curvature of the spine, or pain in the spine. The only disadvantage of X-ray machines is that they emit more intense beams than the machines used for the bone mineral density test.

Why are blood and urine tests useful?

Blood and urine tests are very useful. They make it possible to detect other diseases linked to osteoporosis, such as thyroid gland abnormalities. The most commonly performed tests concern measuring calcium, phosphorus and creatinine blood levels, calcium and creatinine urine levels over a period of 24 hours, urine protein electrophoresis, as well as a red and white blood cell count. Other tests may be carried out, for example the measuring of thyroid hormones. Some of these tests are very useful for evaluating the efficacy of treatment in diagnosed osteoporosis.

The bone mineral density test as a main diagnostic tool

As an essential screening method for osteoporosis, the bone mineral density test provides, above all, information about your bone mineral density, that is, the calcium content of your bones. Your doctor compares this density to a reference value in order to confirm or rule out osteoporosis.

Measuring mineral density

Measuring bone mineral density, or performing the bone mineral density test, allows doctors to evaluate your bones' strength, and indirectly, your risk of osteoporotic fracture. The test is performed especially on the bones which are most frequently affected by osteoporosis, notably the spine, the hip and, less frequently, the wrist. This technique consists of emitting a beam of energy and measuring the remaining energy that passes through bones. The difference between the ingoing and outgoing energy is equal to the amount of energy absorbed. The absorbed energy reflects the bone mineral density: it is higher when the bone density is greater.

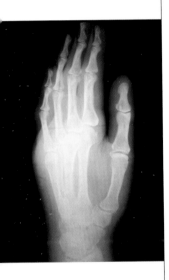

How the test is performed

This simple and painless test takes approximately 15 minutes. You will not need any anesthesia. You will lie down on a table below the test machine. Do not worry, as contrary to other imaging machines, this one does not consist of a tunnel, which may cause anxiety in some patients. You do not need to undress, unless your clothes contain metal objects. Once you are lying down on the table, the test will begin.

Your posture varies according to the bones tested: if your spine is tested, your legs will be raised with the help of a cushion, which flattens the lower part of the spine as much as possible; if, however, your hip is tested, your leg is bound to the table with a strap.

The T-score

In order to interpret the results of the bone mineral density test, your bone mineral density is compared to the average bone density of a young adult of your gender who does not suffer from bone disease : this is the T-score. The T-score reflects your bone mineral density compared to a reference value, which is applicable to your specific population type. The results appear as a standard deviation relative to this reference value. The T-score is generally more negative the older you are.

Interpretation of results

Bone mineral density is normal when it is less than one standard deviation below that of a young adult, that is, a T-score between 0 and -1. When your T-score is between -1 and -2.5, this indicates osteopenia. In concrete terms, this means that you lost between 10 and 25% of your bone mass and that this should be monitored.

When your T-score is ≤-2.5, this indicates osteoporosis. In practice, this means that you have lost more than 25% of your bone mass. On the other hand, if your T-score is ≤ -2.5 and you have had one or several fractures, you suffer from "severe" osteoporosis. Treatment is therefore vital.

The T-score as a statistical value

You should keep in mind that the T-score is a statistical notion. Therefore, a low T-score does not necessarily mean that you will have fractures. For this reason, your doctor also carefully considers your medical history as well as your medical examination before beginning any treatment.

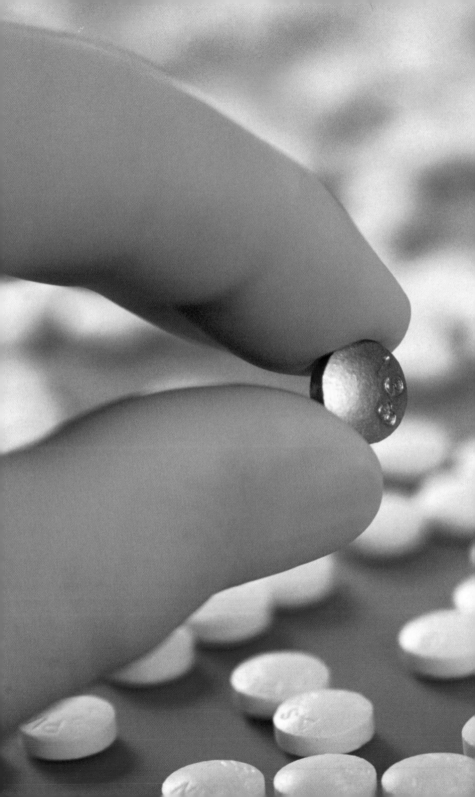

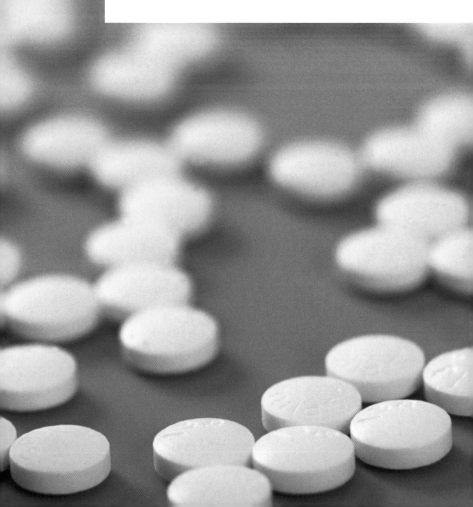

CHAPTER 4:
OSTEOPOROSIS TREATMENT

OSTEOPOROSIS TREATMENT

General measures

Osteoporosis management varies greatly between one case and another. The major aim of treatment is to prevent fractures, which can be extremely unpleasant. Drug treatment for osteoporosis is aimed at improving bone strength so as to reduce the risk of fracture. Treatment differs according to the cause of osteoporosis and depends on each patient's risk of fracture, as evaluated by the doctor.

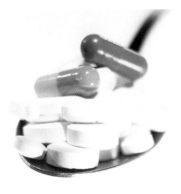

Drug treatment must never overshadow non-drug measures. Preventing falls, for example, is particularly important. The correction of eyesight problems, gait problems and the organization of the patient's home environment must be included in the therapy plan. If you suffer from osteoporosis, it is equally essential that you get regular physical exercise, as this stimulates bone growth.

Available drugs

Different classes of drugs for the treatment of osteoporosis are currently available. Drug treatments can be classified into two large groups, according to their mechanism of action:
• Drugs which inhibit bone resorption, which are also called antiresorptive agents. Calcium, vitamin D, bisphosphonates, raloxifene, calcitonin, estrogens, and estroprogestatives all belong to this class.
• Drugs which stimulate bone growth, which have an anabolic effect. Parathormone is this group's main drug.

Who should get treatment?

Not all osteoporosis sufferers need drug treatment. Starting this type of treatment mainly depends on the T-score obtained from the bone mineral density test. If your T-score, which indicates bone mineral density, is ≤-2.5, your doctor may prescribe an appropriate drug treatment. In fact, a T-score ≤-2.5 is considered to be a major risk for fracture. Nevertheless, bone mineral density only represents risk factors.

When deciding which treatment to prescribe, your doctor must also take other risk factors, especially your age and body weight, into account. Your family history, especially hip fractures in first-degree parents, prolonged immobility, and previous or current corticoid treatment must be taken into account. Your doctor will also take note of any calcium or vitamin D deficiencies and will ask questions about your tobacco and alcohol intake.

Risk factors for falls, for example eyesight or coordination problems, are also important. If you present one or several fragility fractures, that is, fractures not resulting from major trauma, drug treatment is strongly recommended, as you are at very high risk of suffering another fracture.

Treatment possibilities

ANTIRESORPTIVE TREATMENT	BONE GROWTH STIMULATION TREATMENT
• Calcium and vitamin D	• Parathormone
• Estrogens, selective estrogen and estroprogestative receptor modulators, anabolics	• Fluorine (controversial effect)
• Bisphosphonates	• Strontium ranelate (moderate effect)
• Calcitonin	

Calcium

All osteoporosis patients must have sufficient calcium and vitamin D intake. This can be achieved by you diet, but also by drug supplementation. The explanations of this follow below.

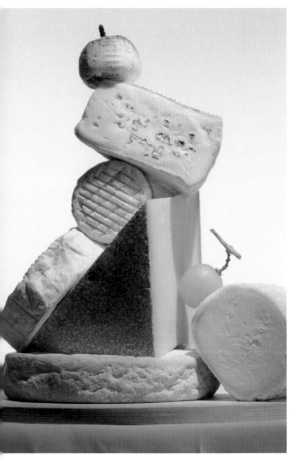

Calcium and vitamins

As it is the main building block of bones, calcium is of utmost importance in the fight against osteoporosis. Its absorption in the digestive tract and its binding to bone tissue largely depend on vitamin D. If you lack vitamin D, less calcium is absorbed by your digestive tract and it will not bind to bone tissue properly.

The main sources of calcium are dairy products and mineral water with a high calcium content. Other dietary sources of calcium include eggs, starches, legumes, meat, fish, etc. Bone tissue contains close to 99% of your body's calcium, whereas only 1% of your body's calcium is found in the blood. The binding of calcium to bone tissue is slowed down if you have a vitamin D and/or K deficiency. Vitamin K, especially that found in meat and liver, activates osteocalcin, a protein found in bones onto which calcium binds itself, and improves this binding. Apart from these dietary sources of vitamin K, there is another source found inside your own body: certain bacteria found in your intestines also produce vitamin K.

Recommended daily allowance of calcium in mg

- Children aged 1 to 3 years: 800
- Children aged 4 to 9 years: 800 – 1 200
- Adolescents: 1 200 – 1 500
- Adults: 900
- Women older than 55 years without HRT: 1 200
- Women older than 55 years with HRT: 1 500
- Men older than 65 years: 1 200

Calcium supplements

Only a balanced diet can enable you to take in the recommended daily allowance of calcium. The majority of experts recommend a daily intake of 1000mg of calcium, which corresponds to approximately one quart of milk. If your diet includes less than 700mg per day, your doctor can prescribe a calcium supplement, which could range from 500mg to 1000mg per day, depending on your needs.

A vitamin D supplement is generally also prescribed to compensate for a lack of sun exposure and improve calcium absorption in your digestive tract. A large selection of calcium-based products is available in pharmacies. Read the labels carefully: calcium content varies greatly between brands. Numerous calcium and vitamin D combinations are also available on the market.

Adverse effects of calcium

An excessive intake of calcium may lead to kidney stones and damage blood vessels. If you suffer from impaired kidney function, an excessive calcium intake is particularly dangerous.

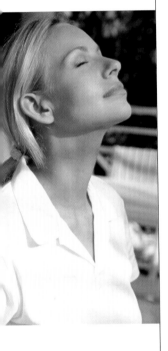

Vitamin D

Vitamin D, which is vital for bone health, plays a key role in metabolizing calcium.

Vitamin D and calcium absorption

The main function of vitamin D is regulating calcium levels in the blood by increasing calcium absorption in the intestines and reducing its excretion through the urine. It is also involved in binding calcium to bone tissue and, should the body need it, depleting it from the bones.

Vitamin D is partly provided by your diet, but your diet alone cannot cover your daily requirements. On average, less than 100 IU of vitamin D is provided by your diet per day, whereas your daily requirement ranges from 400 to 800 IU.

The main sources of vitamin D are oily fish, such as salmon, tuna, sardines, and herring. It can also be found in eggs, meat, and dairy products.

Sun exposure

Apart from dietary sources of vitamin D, the body is able to synthesize vitamin D in the skin under the effect of ultraviolet rays. This is why vitamin D is also called "the sun vitamin". It has been estimated that sun exposure covers 80% to 90% of the body's requirements of vitamin D. Exposing your skin to the sun for 10 to 15 minutes between 11 am and 2 pm, two to three times a week should be sufficient to cover your needs. Elderly people often suffer from a vitamin D deficiency, partly because they do not receive enough sun exposure. When your diet and sun exposure do not cover your needs, a vitamin D drug supplement may be prescribed.

Vitamin D deficiency

A vitamin D deficiency due to an insufficient dietary intake may occur in vegans who do not eat meat, fish, dairy products, or eggs. However, a vitamin D deficiency may also be a result of absorption problems in the intestines, especially in chronic diarrhea due to liver or pancreatic disease. Moreover, it seems that the body's ability to absorb vitamin D in the intestines or to synthesize it under the skin with the effect of ultraviolet rays, decreases with age. This phenomenon is partly responsible for the fact that osteoporosis becomes more frequent with age.

Adverse effects of vitamin D

An excessive vitamin D intake causes hypervitaminosis: surplus vitamin D is stored in the body and becomes toxic. This leads to general disorders, such as loss of appetite, vomiting, diarrhea, drymouth, headaches, increased levels of calcium in the blood, and intense fatigue. Over the long term, calcium deposits in kidneys and vessels have been observed. Vitamin D poisoning is a medical emergency.

Sun exposure and vitamin D requirements

Vitamin D levels are at their lowest in winter. Normal outside activity is sufficient in order to prevent possible winter deficiencies. When this is impossible, your doctor can prescribe a vitamin D supplement in the form of drops, which you must take a few of every day, or in the form of a vial of liquid which you will take every 2 to 6 months.

Bisphosphonates

Bisphosphonates are bone resorption inhibitors: by blocking osteoclast activity, they decrease bone damage. They facilitate the increase in bone mineral density by approximately 5 to 10% and, at the same time, reduce the risk of fracture.

Bisphosphonate action

The bisphosphonate class contains eight substances, notably etidronate, alendronate, and risedronate.

Etidronate is administered in cycles, at a daily dose of 400mg for 14 days, every three months. This is followed by a course of calcium and possibly also vitamin D over the course of 2.5 months. It has been proven that this drug can reduce bone loss after menopause.

Alendronate, prescribed at a continuous daily dose of 10mg, reduces the risk of spine, femur, and radius fractures by approximately 50% after 3 years of treatment. Taking the drug once weekly, at a dose of 70mg, is much more practical and enables you to keep to your treatment more easily.

Risedronate, prescribed at a continuous daily dose of 5mg, reduces the risk of spine fractures by approximately 50% and the risk of hip fractures by a third. It is much more practical for you to take the drug once weekly, as this will allow you to keep to your treatment more easily.

Calcium and vitamin D

Your anti-osteoporotic treatment is most effective if you make sure that you are taking in enough calcium and vitamin D every day. In certain cases, your doctor may decide to prescribe supplements to go along with other treatments.

How should bisphosphonates be taken?

All bisphosphonates are in the form of tablets, which should be swallowed on an empty stomach, with a glass of water, as they are very poorly absorbed, and therefore ineffective, when taken with food. After having taken the drug, do not lie down, but rather remain in a vertical position for at least 30 minutes, so that the drug does not rise back up in the esophagus, which could cause damage. If your doctor prescribes calcium and vitamin D as a parallel treatment, they should be taken at least 2 hours after the bisphosphonates, as they could reduce the absorption of bisphosphonates. Bisphosphonates must generally be taken during at least 4 years. If you suffer a fracture during this period and if you have been taking the drug according to the prescription, your doctor may consider a different treatment.

Adverse effects of bisphosphonates

Bisphosphonates are generally well-tolerated. However, they can sometimes lead to gastrointestinal problems, such as diarrhea, nausea, and abdominal pain. Fever and headaches may also occur. In rare cases, bisphosphonates have caused skin reactions, abnormally decreased calcium levels in the blood, and bone tissue death in the jaw, which is called osteonecrosis.

Drug treatment is not the only answer

Whether you are undergoing drug treatment or not, your lifestyle also plays a key role in managing your osteoporosis. If you suffer from osteoporosis, you should get regular physical exercise in order to strengthen your bones and improve balance and coordination, thereby reducing the risk of falling and fracturing your bones. Preventing falls also entails adopting certain habits and making a few changes in the organization of your home environment.

Drugs for the treatment of postmenopausal osteoporosis

During menopause, the production of estrogens diminishes, leading to bone loss, which may cause osteoporosis. More than one out of three women are at risk of developing this condition. Treatments, such as bisphosphonates or calcitonin could be very effective, however, it is sometimes a good idea to tackle the problem at its source and counteract the lack of estrogens.

Hormone replacement therapy

Hormone replacement therapy (HRT), which often combines estrogen and progesterone, compensate for reduced estrogen levels resulting from menopause. They are often prescribed for alleviating climacteric problems like hot flashes and mood swings, which affect many menopausal women. These drugs have also been shown to reduce the risk of fracture. At present, there is sufficient clinical data supporting the theory that estrogen or estroprogestative treatments are an effective way of preventing bone loss. Such treatments even seem to increase bone mass in women around the time of menopause!

HRT and osteoporotic fractures

It is not usual practice to prescribe HRT to osteoporotic women who have never had this type of therapy before. If, however, the patient has low bone mineral density and other risk factors for fracture, her doctor may consider HRT.

In fact, data from a series of clinical studies confirms that HRT leads to fewer osteoporotic fractures. The treatment's protective effect is believed to be particularly pronounced in women who start hormone therapy 3 to 5 years after menopause. A reduction in the occurrence of spinal compression has been observed from the first year of treatment.

Adverse effects of HRT

These treatments, especially if they are started in older women, could however lead to harmless adverse effects, such as weight gain, water retention, etc. More serious adverse effects have been observed in the cardiovascular system, for example, the occurrence of phlebitis. Another negative aspect of HRT is that it increases the risk of breast cancer by 30% after 15 years of regular treatment. This is why the doctor has to evaluate the benefits of such treatments on a case-by-case basis. Therefore, if your doctor considers the risks of HRT too high in your particular case, he or she will prescribe a different treatment. In all cases, treatment will always be limited to a certain period of time and will be prescribed at the lowest possible dose.

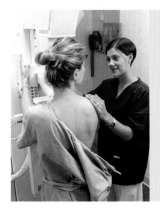

HRT and breast cancer

Today, there is proof that short term estrogen therapy, that is less than 5 years, does not increase the risk of breast cancer. On the other hand, if HRT lasts longer than 10 years, the risk of breast cancer seems to increase slightly. There is not yet any sufficient clinical data allowing us to make conclusions about the link between estroprogestative treatment and the risk of breast cancer. Nevertheless, numerous studies seem to suggest that the risk is the same during estroprogestative treatment.

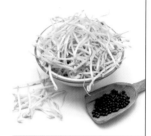

Other treatments for postmenopausal osteoporosis

Tamoxifen is currently used in the treatment of breast cancer and stimulates the skeleton's estrogenic receptors. According to certain studies, this drug seems to reduce bone loss, but it is not officially authorized for the treatment of osteoporosis.

Are phytoestrogens effective?

Phytoestrogens are plant substances which are claimed to have a similar action as that of estrogens. They occur naturally in certain vegetables, such as soy, and are also available as over-the-counter dietary supplements. These substances are therefore not evaluated in the same way as drugs are before being put on the market. Although they could have a positive effect on certain symptoms of menopause, they can in no way substitute osteoporosis drug treatments. It is therefore better to leave it up to your doctor to choose the most appropriate treatment.

What is a SERM ?

Tamoxifen is a SERM (Selective Estrogen Receptor Modulator). Strictly speaking, these drugs are not actually hormones. They act differently, depending on the organ in question. Their effects on bones and vessels are similar to those of estrogens, while their effect on the uterus and breasts are opposite to that of estrogens. Much like estrogens, they slightly increase the risk of phlebitis, however, they do not relieve hot flashes and other menopause-related subjective problems.

Raloxifene is sold in the United States under several different brand names.

Raloxifene

Raloxifene decreases bone loss by stimulating estrogen receptors in bone tissue. This way, bone mass increases and the risk of spine fractures decreases in menopausal women suffering from

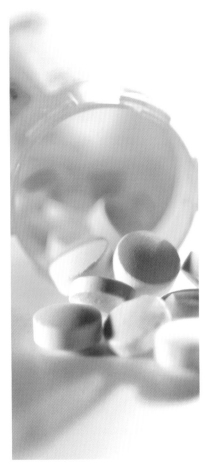

osteoporosis. However, it does not seem to reduce the risk of other fractures.

As raloxifene has no impact on climacteric problems, it cannot replace HRT treatment in this respect. On the other hand, raloxifene is used increasingly in the management of postmenopausal osteoporosis, because it seems to reduce the risk of breast cancer, despite the fact that it also increases the risk of venous thrombosis. Contrary to estrogen taken as a hormone replacement, raloxifene has no negative effect on endometriosis. Studies also demonstrated that this drug reduces bad cholesterol and the risk of heart attack or stroke.

The drug is in the form of tablets, which must be taken daily. In general, treatment stretches over several years. Its main adverse effects are hot flashes, leg cramps, and an increased risk of venous thrombosis. For this reason, raloxifene is not recommended if you have a history of phlebitis.

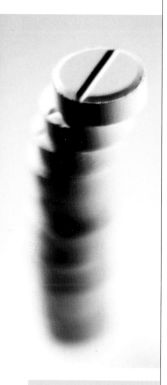

Other available treatments

Most drugs used for the treatment of osteoporosis act by blocking bone resorption. Just like estrogens, estroprogestatives, SERM, calcium, and vitamin D, calcitonin also has a direct effect on resorption. Strontium has a dual action: it inhibits bone resorption while also stimulating bone growth.

Calcitonin

This hormone is usually produced in parathyroid glands and blocks bone resorption by acting directly on osteoclasts. Calcitonin has been proven effective in the prevention of spine fractures. In addition, it has an analgesic effect and is therefore also prescribed for relieving pain caused by spine fractures.

The main adverse effects of calcitonin taken subcutaneously or intramuscularly at a dose of 50 to 100 IU once a day, are digestive problems, such as nausea, abdominal pain and hot flashes. Calcitonin nasal spray, at a daily dose of 200 IU, has fewer adverse effects. In certain cases, calcitonin loses its effectiveness after a certain treatment time.

Why strontium ranelate is exceptional

Strontium is a heavier mineral than calcium. It is absorbed in the intestines and has a strong affinity for bone tissue, where it partially substitutes calcium. Strontium is exceptional mainly because

The analgesic effect of calcitonin

As calcitonin has an analgesic effect, it is especially used to relieve severe pain resulting from spinal compression fractures.

it has a dual action: it increases bone growth and, at the same time, reduces bone resorption. Several clinical studies demonstrated a significantly reduced risk of fracture in menopausal women. A protective effect against fractures has even been observed in persons older than 80 years.

Adverse effects, such as diarrhea, nausea, and headaches at the beginning of treatment have been observed in clinical studies. These adverse effects disappeared after 3 months of treatment.

In practice, strontium ranelate is taken at a daily dose of 2g, as a soluble granules contained in sachets. The granules must be taken 2 hours after dinner or calcium supplements, as calcium and food decrease the product's absorption. The treatment time is at least 36 months.

Drug combinations

In severe osteoporosis cases, doctors may decide to prescribe a combination of drugs with different modes of action in order to combine the anti osteoporotic effects of each drug. For example, HRT can be successfully combined with a bisphosphonate. Similarly, the combination of raloxifene and a bisphosphonate is a winner. The combination of raloxifene and HRT, however, is contra-indicated.

Contra-indications of strontium

As strontium contains galactose and lactose, the drug is contra-indicated in patients suffering from galactose malabsorption or lactase deficiency.

It is also contra-indicated in patients with impaired kidney function, which is defined by a creatinine clearance of less than 30 mL/min.

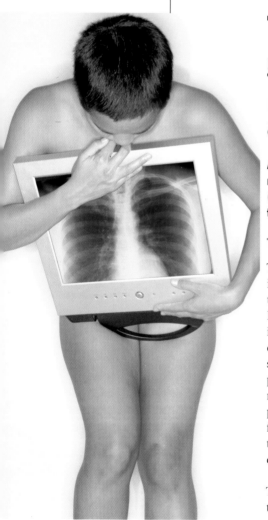

The bone growth drugs parathormone and fluorine

Among the currently available treatments, only the parathyroid hormone (PTH), fluorine, and partially also strontium, increase bone growth.

Teriparatide

Teriparatide, a bone growth agent, is derived from the human parathormone, using biotechnology. It stimulates bone growth by increasing the number and action of osteoblasts. In a large clinical study on menopausal women, teriparatide, at a daily dose of 20µg, reduced the percentage of patients presenting new spinal compression fractures by 65%. At the same time, the risk of non-spinal fractures decreased by 77%.

The product is especially prescribed to women with severe osteoporosis.

Doctors may also prescribe teriparatide treatment to women who do not tolerate or do not respond to other available products. This treatment is often combined with calcium and vitamin D supplements. The most common adverse effects, which are generally light or moderate, include cramps in the lower limbs, nausea, and headaches. A slight increase in calcium levels in the blood has been observed in the hours following the injection.

In practice, the patient takes teriparatide subcutaneously by injecting herself every day with a pen already containing 28 days worth of treatment. At present, treatment time is limited to 18 months.

An instruction manual for calcium fluoride

Fluorine must be taken with calcium-free water. If you eat or drink dairy-based food or beverages, you must take fluorine either half an hour before or 2 hours after the meal.

Fluorine

The use of fluorine dates back a long time. Its mechanism of action is based on bone growth which is stimulated by osteoblasts. It has been established that the use of fluorine leads to an increase in bone mineral density, particularly in the lumbar vertebrae. However, it has not yet been determined whether it reduces spinal compression fractures.

Certain studies seem to suggest that fluorine could increase the risk of other fractures, which could be the result of the poor quality of newly-formed bone tissue. In practice, fluorine is taken every day at a dose of 50mg of calcium fluoride. The product must be taken between meals and a considerable time before or after taking a calcium supplement, with calcium-free water.

A calcium supplement, and if needed, a vitamin D supplement, must be combined with the treatment. Fluorine treatment should not be proposed to patients older than 70 years.

Contra-indications of teriparatide

Teriparatide is contra-indicated in patients with an increased level of calcium in the blood, severely impaired kidney function, or a bone disease other than osteoporosis. The drug should not be taken during pregnancy or breastfeeding. Women who have a history of kidney stones should be careful when using this drug.

Anabolic steroids

Anabolic steroids, which are similar to testosterone, are sometimes used for treating diagnosed osteoporosis in menopausal women. Nandrolone decanoate is part of this class of drugs and is available in vials containing 50mg/mL of nandrolone decanoate.

As this treatment must be administered for a long period in postmenopausal osteoporosis, it often causes the appearance of androgenic signs, such as excess body hair. Therefore, this product is only very rarely used in women.

Osteoporosis and phytotherapy

Certain plants may be a valuable natural alternative for osteoporosis treatment and prevention. However, you should take note of the fact that, like any other treatment, plants with medicinal properties must only be taken under close monitoring in order to avoid overdosing or using them incorrectly. Remember that "natural" does not mean "safe".

Beneficial plants for osteoporosis patients

The main benefit of plants such as field horsetail, nettle, and alfalfa for the treatment and prevention of osteoporosis is essentially their remineralizing properties.

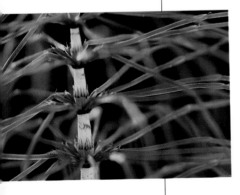

• **Field horsetail (*Equisetum arvense*)** Also known as common horsetail, this perennial plant belongs to the Equisetacae family and grows in the moist soils in all corners of the world, except Australia. Horsetail has a 35cm-high fertile stem, over which towers a 60cm-high sterile stem. While it has no flowers, it contains spikes that resemble needles. The therapeutic benefit of this plant lies in its high content in minerals, particularly silica, which promotes the regrowth of connective tissue and the binding of calcium to bones. Moreover, horsetail also contains magnesium and potassium. It is also said to prevent osteoporosis and improve the healing of bone fractures. Only the sterile stem of horsetail, whether dried or fresh, is used. For osteoporosis, it is only used in the form of capsules which contain dry powder or extract, or as an infused brew, juice, or drops which can be bought at the pharmacy.

• **Alfalfa (*Medicago sativa*)**
Alfalfa, or lucerne, is a herbaceous perennial plant which grows in meadows, wildlands, and on cultivated land. Measuring 70cm in height, the stem of this plant carries flowers in colors ranging from yellow to purple, forming clusters. Alfalfa is very rich in protein but also in vitamins and minerals, including calcium, as well as trace elements such as ion,

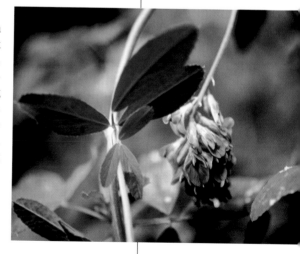

phosphorus, silica, and magnesium, which give the plant its remineralizing properties. Moreover, this plant also contains the plant estrogen coumestrol, which can be useful for treating menopause problems and osteoporosis. Alfalfa is available in the form of capsules, drops which must be diluted, and liquid extracts, but can also be consumed as a herbal tea.

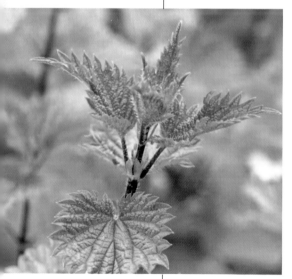

• **Nettle (*Urtica dioica and Urtica urens*)**
The numerous benefits of nettle, especially its diuretic and anti-inflammatory effects, have been recognized for centuries. Nettle also has a remineralizing property. Much like field horsetail, it contains large amounts of minerals, such as potassium, silica, and magnesium. These minerals are found in nettle leaves, which can be consumed as tea, although nettle capsules are also available on the market.

• **Spiny bamboo (*Bambusa arundinacea*)**
Spiny bamboo is a fast-growing perennial plant from the Poacea family. It is found in Asia and is widely used in India and China for its medicinal properties. Its stem is rich in silica, which has remineralizing properties. In the United States, this plant is available in the form of capsules made from a bamboo stem extract.

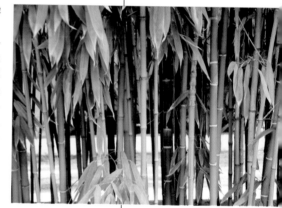

Field horsetail and marsh horsetail

It is absolutely vital not to confuse field horsetail with marsh horsetail (Equisetum palustre), which contains toxic alkaloids that may be very dangerous. If you pick horsetail in meadows, show the plants to a botanist or herbalist before consuming them.

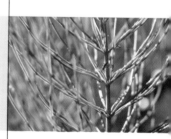

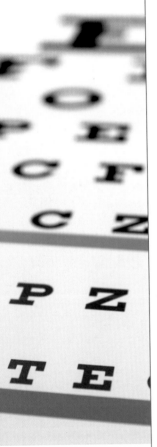

Preventing falls

In osteoporosis patients, even a light impact may cause fracture. It is therefore vital to protect your weakened bones by eliminating all risk factors for falls. These factors are found everywhere, but it is easy to rectify them.

Correct your eyesight

Age and the deterioration of eyesight often go hand in hand, much like poor eyesight and the risk of falling. Avoid falling by having your eyesight checked regularly. Should your ophthalmologist prescribe glasses or contact lenses, wear them all the time, from the moment you wake up.

Walk with firm steps

Put your stilettos back in the closet! Rather wear shoes with flat or low heels, which are comfortable and provide good support. Choose a pair with anti-slip soles.

To make it easier for you to walk, you can also use a cane, which improves your stability. Make sure that it is the correct height and regularly check the condition of the rubber tip.

Organize your home environment

Start by clearing all rooms in your home of objects which might cause you to fall, such as extension cables, inconveniently placed slippery carpets, plants, etc. When it comes to the floor, you should absolutely ban all slippery materials like tiles or waxed wooden floors, on which you could easily slip.

Good lighting is essential. Install lamps everywhere in your home and do not forget to switch them on should you get up at night.

A good number of falls occur in staircases. Therefore, you should make sure that they are as safe as possible for you to use. Install railings on each side of the staircase and, most importantly, do not wax them if they are made out of wood.

Also remember to make your bathroom and toilet safe rooms: install support rails and do not forget to put an anti-slip mat in your shower or bath.

Be careful of certain substances

Certain drugs are known to impair alertness. Sleeping pills, tranquilizers, and other sedatives are examples of such drugs. You should avoid taking them as best as you can. Even if they have been prescribed to you by your doctor, discuss possible alternatives with him.

Alcohol also causes falls and, moreover, is harmful to bone tissue. Osteoporosis and alcohol are therefore not a good combination. You must reduce your alcohol consumption.

Hip protectors

External hip protectors are made of foam or semi-rigid shells inside a special pair of briefs. Should you fall, these protectors will absorb some of the impact and efficiently prevent your femoral head from fracturing. Although they are not very attractive, they can be very useful to osteoporosis patients, to whom a fracture could be very dangerous.

The occupational therapist's role

It can sometimes be difficult to recognize all the hazards in one's home. Therefore, why not consult an occupational therapist? This health professional will come to your home and evaluate the risks of falling and suggest making certain changes. If you do not know any occupational therapists, your doctor will be able to recommend one.

Treatment of fractures

For osteoporosis patients, fractures are unfortunately a part of daily life. However, contrary to what many people think, osteoporosis does not impair bone regrowth. The bone can fuse back together, but only if the fracture is treated correctly.

Wrist fractures

When falling, one often tries to break the fall with one's hand. The wrist is therefore bearing the entire body weight, and a fracture occurs. It is painful, swells

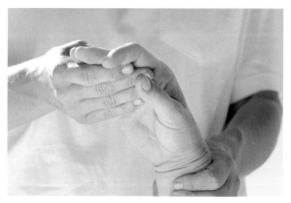

and the person finds it difficult to move their wrist. In simple fractures, where the bone has not pierced the skin, an orthopedic treatment is appropriate: after realigning the two broken ends of the bone, the wrist is put in a cast, which the patient must keep on until the bones have completely fused back together.

In comminuted fractures, when the bone has fractured in several places, surgery is necessary. The procedure consists of realigning the ends of bones and maintaining them in this position with a screw plate or pins. After the operation, the wrist is immobilized with a cast or splint.

Fractures of the femoral head

Due to its kinked shape, the femoral head is a particularly fragile bone. When it fractures, the patient feels severe pain in the hip and is unable to walk or even lift the leg.

The first treatment phase often involves surgery. The surgeon may decide to place a partial or complete hip prosthesis. This solution is often the first choice for the elderly. In younger and more active patients, osteosynthesis may be performed: after putting the bones back into place, the surgeon stabilizes them with a long nail and screws.

In all cases, surgery is followed by a period of immobilization where the patient must avoid stepping on the leg for several months. Elderly patient care must be particularly meticulous. Complications from forced bed rest include bedsores, phlebitis, and pulmonary embolism.

Bedsores

Bedsores, which result from bed confinement, are a common complication of hip fractures in the elderly. Many cases of bedsores only heal after months, or even years, of treatment. To patients, they are a great burden to bear, because the severe pain, threat of septicemia, and the risk of complications drastically lower the quality of patients' lives.

According to scientific publications, 80% of all bedsores occur in the pelvis and heels. Moreover, the danger of bedsores increases with the patient's degree of immobility. Bedsores are more dangerous when the patient has completed the period of bed rest, and for example, he or she loses consciousness or needs anesthesia. It is also important to stress that patient care has an effect on immobilization. During the daytime, patient care involves changing the patient's position, whereas the night time is a still period, presenting a greater risk of bedsores. This is why bedsores usually arise at night.

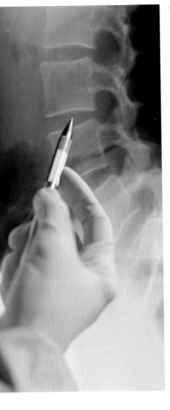

Treatment of spine fractures

The treatment of spine fractures is above all medical, consisting of bed rest and pain killers. In very painful spinal compression fractures which do not respond to drug treatment, vertebroplasty and kyphoplasty can be useful.

Spine fractures

Spine fractures, or spinal compression fractures, are often a sign of osteoporosis. This type of fracture may be caused by a simple accidental move. A vertebra collapses and becomes compressed between two other vertebrae. Whether or not this is painful depends on the affected vertebra, sometimes there is no pain at all. The most commonly affected vertebrae include dorsal and lumbar vertebrae. Cervical vertebrae are affected much more rarely. A decrease in the person's height is very characteristic of spinal compression fractures. Sometimes, this type of fracture can lead to back deformation.

Medical treatment

The aims of the treatment include prevention of future vertebral collapse, pain relief, and the return to a normal lifestyle. In the beginning, bed rest is often necessary for relieving pain. For the same purpose, the doctor may prescribe analgesics and non-steroidal anti-inflammatories, or inject calcitonin. As these injections may cause nausea, vomiting, and hot flashes, an antimimetic agent may be necessary. When pain has subsided and the patient can resume his or her usual daily activities, wearing a back brace may sometimes be necessary. Although they do not prevent back deformation, back braces bring pain relief and allow patients to resume their daily activities more quickly. Back braces are however only useful for vertebral fractures in the lower back. In addition, patients must undergo physiotherapy and kinesitherapy.

Vertebroplasty

Vertebroplasty consists in injecting a resin with the consistency of toothpaste into the compressed vertebra. This injection is performed under the control of X-ray and CT machines. The resin hardens within a few minutes, and by strengthening the vertebra, it acts mechanically on the pain caused by the fracture. Certain highly-experienced radiologists can treat several vertebrae at he same time, under the same anesthesia. This is done for very painful spinal compression fractures.

Kyphoplasty

More and more frequently, orthopedic surgeons propose kyphoplasty when medication is unable to stop pain. This method consists in first inserting a small inflatable balloon into the vertebra, and then inflating it until the vertebra regains its normal shape and the compressed area straightens. The balloon is then taken out and a repairing cement is injected into the cavity. The same indications apply for kyphoplasty as for vertebroplasty.

Non-steroidal anti-inflammatories

Low doses of non-steroidal anti-inflammatories reduce pain and lower fever. In higher doses, they have an anti-inflammatory effect.

Taking these substances may lead to severe or light adverse effects in the digestive system, such as acid reflux disease, nausea, ulcers, and digestive hemorrhage. In order to reduce the occurrence of adverse effects, you must adhere to the dose and treatment time that your doctor prescribed.

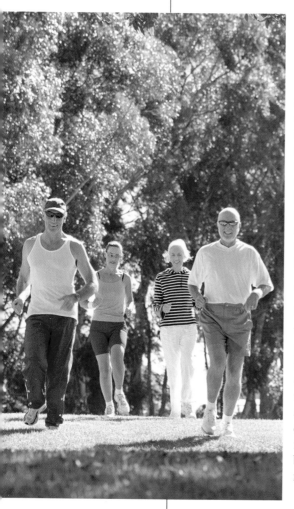

Physical activity

Contrary to popular belief, bone disease does not excuse one from engaging in regular physical activity. On the contrary, physical movement is an important part of osteoporosis management. Nevertheless, before starting a sport, ask your doctor for advice, as he or she is the best person to evaluate your ability to practice a sport regularly.

The many virtues of physical activity

When you engage in a regular physical activity, your skeleton is subject to certain mechanical constraints. By acting against these constraints, the bones that are used strengthen. However, exercise is only beneficial if it is practiced regularly, because bones gradually weaken when no longer used.

Apart from improving bone strength, exercise improves balance and coordination in the elderly, which in turn helps reduce the risk of falling.

Which are the most appropriate sports?

The most beneficial sports for osteoporosis are those that work the supporting joints, particularly those in the spine and legs. Therefore, walking, running, and dancing are perfect for osteoporosis patients. Walking is of even greater benefit if done at a fast pace.

Even certain sports that do not work the supporting joints are beneficial for osteoporosis cases. This includes weight training, which can help strengthen the bones if the muscle contraction is sustained.

Although they have no direct impact on the bones, sports like stretching and yoga ensure good posture, teach correct breathing, and improve flexibility.

Although swimming does not require you to support your entire body weight, it may be particularly useful if

Hydrotherapy and mineral springs

Neither hydrotherapy nor mineral springs can cure osteoporosis. They may, however, help relieve pain due to fracture. Hot springs are especially effective for pain relief.

you have previously suffered from spinal compression fractures, as it reduces pain and prevents hunching. If you have a hunched back, it is better to swim on your back.

While many sports are beneficial for osteoporosis patients, sports that might cause you to fall should be avoided. Cycling, especially if it is done on slippery or rough terrain, and skiing should be considered off-limits. Sports that involve excessive strain, such as heavy weightlifting, are also not appropriate, as they could lead to spinal fractures.

Physiotherapy and kinesitherapy

Your doctor may prescribe physiotherapy or kinesitherapy sessions as a rehabilitation treatment or simply to prevent further fractures. During these session, you will learn the exercises that are right for you. Once you have completed the sessions, you should continue doing these exercises. Massages can also help you to alleviate pain following fracture.

Sit up straight!

Good body posture helps osteoporosis patients to better follow their daily activities and to reduce pain. No matter what you are doing, keep your back straight, tuck in your tummy and chin and keep your shoulders back.

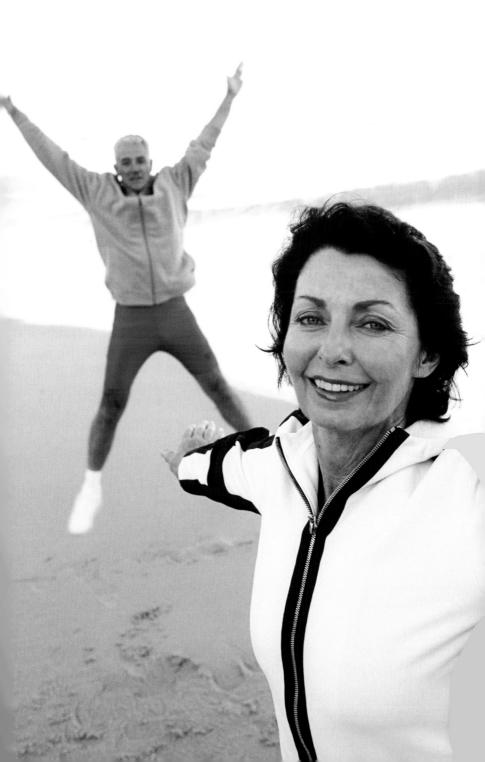

MISCONCEPTIONS ABOUT OSTEOPOROSIS

Although osteoporosis is a common condition, there are many misunderstandings about this disease.

Osteoporosis is painful

Osteoporosis is a silent and painless disease. It is not osteoporosis itself that is painful, but in fact the secondary fractures due to a fall or accidental move which cause pain. The most common fractures occur in the spine, wrist or hip. In order to prevent fractures, avoid all activities that might cause you to fall or make any accidental moves. Should you fracture your wrist or a vertebra, there are numerous effective pain treatments available.

If you drink a lot of milk, you are safe from osteoporosis

The calcium contained in dairy products is one of the main factors influencing bone mass. However, the consumption of dairy products cannot single-handedly prevent osteoporosis. Tobacco, alcohol, a sedentary lifestyle, as well as overexercising, a lack of sun exposure and certain genetic factors can also make you vulnerable to osteoporosis. Remember that milk is not the food with the highest calcium content: cheese and yogurt contain much more.

Osteoporosis only affects adults

Osteoporosis mostly affects menopausal women, when estrogen secretion decreases. However, osteoporosis can also affect children and adolescents. Osteoporosis in children is often linked to a chronic disease, such as chronic intestinal inflammation (Crohn's disease).

It may also result from long-term corticoid treatment, as in severe cases of asthma, for example. In adolescents, several factors can be responsible for osteoporosis: smoking, numerous problems and deficiencies linked to anorexia, drastic weight-loss diets low in essential nutrients such as calcium, or excessively intense physical activity, especially high-level sports.

Meat is good for your bones

When you eat meat, you are providing your body with essential amino acids which it needs in order to function normally. Too much meat, however, is actually bad for your bones. During digestion, meat is broken down into acids, which are stored in your body and then excreted.

In order to neutralize these acidic substances, your body must use the alkaline substances, such as calcium, that are found in our bones. Over the long term, eating too much meat will contribute to the body's acidification, depleting your bones of minerals and making them more vulnerable to osteoporosis.

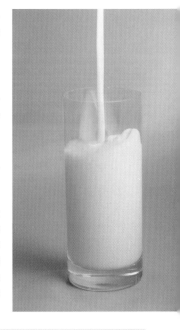

Osteoporosis and cancer

Cancer and osteoporosis may be linked, but this is not always the case. A prostate cancer patient may develop osteoporosis due to the treatment (androgen blockage) for his prostate cancer. Similarly, a women suffering from breast cancer may develop osteoporosis as a result of the anti-estrogen treatment that she receives for her breast cancer. The opposite can also be true: certain osteoporosis treatments can increase the risk of developing certain cancers. For example, long-term HRT slightly increases the risk of breast cancer. Apart from these specific cases, however, there is no link between osteoporosis and cancer.

THE ANSWERS TO YOUR QUESTIONS

Why are more women affected by osteoporosis than men?

The activity of osteoclasts and osteoblasts depends on several factors, including sex hormones. In women, these hormones are closely involved in bone mass evolution. Around the age of 50, sex hormone levels in the blood drop in women, which is referred to as menopause. This hormone decrease is associated often associated with climacteric symptoms, such as hot flashes, mood swings, or weight gain. As far as bones are concerned, osteoclast activity becomes predominant, resulting in bone loss and possibly osteoporosis.

Is osteoporosis hereditary?

Osteoporosis itself is not a hereditary condition: there is no osteoporosis gene. However, bone mineral density is influenced by genetic factors. If you suffer from osteoporosis, your children may be predisposed to develop this condition, too. Indeed, clinical trials have demonstrated that bone mineral mass of children whose parents have osteoporosis is lower than those of other children. However, there is no need for alarm: there are steps you can take to help prevent osteoporosis. Getting enough calcium and vitamin D, along with regular physical exercise, lower your child's risk for osteoporosis, too.

Is osteoporosis painful?

Osteoporosis is a progressive and silent disease. It is not a painful disease in itself: pain only arises when you fracture a bone. Wrist fractures are particularly painful when wrist bones have not properly fused back together, leading to wrist deformation. Hip fractures are extremely painful and most often require surgical treatment. Spinal compression fractures may also cause strong pain, especially in the mid and lower back. Thanks to medical advances, this pain can be relieved using several effective treatments.

I am overweight. Am I more likely to develop osteoporosis?

The answer is no. Factors which can predispose you to osteoporosis include a short stature and low body weight. On the contrary, excess weight seems to protect against osteoporosis. Nevertheless, it is important to notice that estrogen decline related to menopause plays a far more important role in the occurrence of osteoporosis than body weight, although the latter has many other harmful effects on your health. Therefore, it is vital to eat a balanced diet, whatever your body weight, and to exercise regularly in order to prevent osteoporosis.

What is the role of physical activity in preventing osteoporosis?

Physical activity plays a crucial role in preventing osteo-porosis. Individuals who lead a sedentary lifestyle are more prone to develop osteoporosis than those who are physically active. When you engage in physical exercise, two kinds of forces are applied on your bones: compression and traction. During physical activity, the weight of the body exerts the force of compression on bones, whereas contracting muscles exert a traction force on bones. To resist to this stress, bones become stronger. Without regular stress, they become weaker. Yet, the best way to prevent and treat osteoporosis is to maintain bone mass. Therefore, make a point of exercising regularly in order to slow down bone loss and stay healthy.

Does osteodensitometry present any risks?

In order to measure bone density, osteodensitometry uses X-rays, much like conventional X-rays. Radiation produced by the osteodensitometer is much weaker than that produced by an X-ray machine. Therefore, there is no risk of radiation poisoning. However, there are some contra-indications, notably pregnancy, as X-rays can be harmful to the fetus. Moreover, osteo-densitometry cannot be performed if you were admi-nistered an injection containing a radioactive product, e.g. for a bone scan, or a barium sulfate contrast medium 2-3 days before the test.

Can I cure my osteoporosis if I change my diet?

Although a sufficient intake of calcium and vitamin D, along with a good acid-base balance, helps stabilize bone mass, it is impossible to fully recover the bone mass that you have lost throughout your life. Although diet cannot cure osteoporosis, it can slow down bone loss.

I have osteoporosis. Must I cut out salt?

No, it is not necessary to completely cut salt from your diet. When consumed in moderation, salt contains essential minerals for your body. However, an excessive salt intake increases the level of calcium excreted through the urine. A hormone known as parathormone seems to be responsible for this phenomenon. Therefore, do not add too much salt to your dishes. Some more advice: Cheese, crackers, cold cuts, prepared sauces, and ready-made dishes should be eaten sparingly. When cooking, use herbs and spices to enhance the flavor of your dishes instead of adding more salt. At the supermarket, carefully read product labels and do not buy high-sodium food (note that 400mg of sodium are equivalent to 1g of salt).

I am lactose-intolerant. What can I eat instead of dairy products to consume the recommended daily allowance in calcium?

Many other foods and beverages contain calcium, starting with mineral water: some brands of water contain more 500mg/L of calcium. You can also find calcium-enriched soy milk that contains the same amount of calcium as milk. With respect to foods, canned fish like salmon and sardines are also good sources of calcium, as are certain legumes like dried beans or lentils. Do not forget fruit and vegetables, such as broccoli and dried figs. Although the calcium content of these foods is not as high as that of dairy products, having a varied diet will help you to get sufficient amounts of calcium.

Will I put on weight if I eat too much calcium?

No, calcium in itself is not fattening. However, some high-calcium foods also contain large amounts of fats or sugars, which will make you gain weight. Therefore, opt for low-calorie products, so that you get sufficient calcium without putting on weight. For instance, yogurt and skim milk contain far fewer calories than cheese. Even if their calcium contents are lower, vegetables like cabbage and spinach are another suitable option, which will not make you overweight.

Which foods contain vitamin D?

Approximately 10% of the recommended daily allowance of vitamin D is covered by diet. Vitamin D is mostly found in egg yolk, dairy products such as butter and cheese, offal, and oily fish such as herring, salmon, and sardine. However, note that almost 90% of the vitamin D you need is produced in the skin by the action of UVB rays from the sun. Therefore, it is essential that you expose your skin to the sun every day, for about 15 minutes, if possible.

Are there precautions to take when undergoing bisphosphonate treatments?

If taken orally, bisphosphonates are poorly absorbed by the digestive tract: Only 3% of the dose is assimilated. In order to prevent impaired absorption, wait at least 4 hours after meals to take the pills. If you are also taking calcium and vitamin D supplements at the same time, wait at least 2 hours after taking the bisphosphonate to take your supplements. Remain in an upright position for 30 minutes after having taken the bisphosphonate pills. This way, you are preventing the drug from rising back up in your esophagus, which could cause irritation and damage. For the same reason, do not chew the tablet or let it dissolve in your mouth; swallow it with a glass of water. Should you have difficulty swallowing or if you feel any pain behind the breast bone, inform your doctor. He or she might need to prescribe a different treatment.

CONCLUSION

This guide provides you with information on osteoporosis, attempts to answer some of the questions you may have, and also addresses disease prevention.

• **Who is osteoporosis prevention aimed at?** Prevention measures are particularly beneficial to all people who are likely to develop secondary osteoporosis stemming from certain medical conditions or treatments. Nobody should take osteoporosis lightly since we are all to some extent at risk for developing this disease.

• **How can we prevent osteoporosis?** Regular physical activity from childhood on helps build a strong bone mass. Ideally, even after adolescence, people should exercise enough to slow down bone loss. Furthermore, smoking should be stopped and alcohol should be consumed in moderation. Another priority is to consume sufficient calcium and vitamin D throughout your life.

• **Should postmenopausal women systematically be screened for osteoporosis?** It is not a general rule to perform a bone mineral density test on each woman at the onset of menopause. Nevertheless, some experts recommend it in women who present other risk factors.

Clinical trials have shown that postmenopausal osteoporosis could be delayed using hormone replacement therapy. Although HRT is primarily prescribed to relieve menopause symptoms, it has been proven to reduce bone resorption. However, the protection against osteoporotic fractures conferred by HRT seems to lessen with time. Moreover, HRT presents some drawbacks, notably a slightly increased risk of breast cancer. For this reason, the decision to start such a treatment must be made case by case, after having weighed the pros and the cons.

• **Are there alternatives to HRT?** Bisphosphonates and calcitonin are two other options. Many clinical trials have underlined their preventive effects on fractures and vertebral collapse in postmenopausal women.

The treatment of senile osteoporosis essentially aims to preserve bone mass, prevent falls, and relieve pain, particularly in case of vertebral collapse. Calcium and vitamin D supplements must be prescribed if necessary. Other measures can be considered, such as use of bisphosphonates, beginning an anabolic treatment, etc.

We hope that reading this book has helped you to better understand osteoporosis and that you will be able to prevent it or, if need be, to make the appropriate treatment decisions for you.

GLOSSARY

ANTIOXIDANTS: Molecules which reduce the harmful impact of free radicals on the body.

ATHEROSCLEROSIS: Condition characterized by the accumulation of cholesterol-rich fatty deposits in the inner walls of medium- and large-sized arteries. These deposits restrict the flow of blood to the heart, brain, and tissues, which may lead to heart attack or stroke.

BODY MASS INDEX: International standard for weight measurement. It can be obtained by dividing your weight in pounds times 703 by your height in inches squared, or dividing your weight in kilograms by your height in meters squared. Normal values range between 18.5 and $25kg/m^2$.

BONE MINERAL DENSITY (BMD): Measure of the amount of minerals contained in a defined volume of bone. BMD is expressed in g/cm^2.

CALCEMIA: Level of calcium in the blood. Normally, this level remains stable, close to 2.5 millimoles per liter of blood.

CIRRHOSIS: Chronic liver disease in which normal liver cells are replaced by scar tissue.

CROHN'S DISEASE: Chronic inflammatory disease of the intestines. It mainly causes chronic diarrhea, often associated with abdominal pain.

CUSHING'S DISEASE: Rare condition resulting from an overproduction of cortisol by the adrenal glands or by prolonged cortisone use.

ESTROGEN: Hormone produced by the ovaries, which is involved in the development and maintenance of female features (particularly the breasts). Elevated estrogen blood levels induce ovulation.

ACID REFLUX DISEASE: Condition where the stomach's acidic contents flow back into the esophagus because of a lower esophageal sphincter dysfunction.

HORMONE-DEPENDENT CANCER: Cancer whose growth is promoted by certain hormones. Prostate, breast, and endometrial cancers may be hormone-dependent.

HYPOGONADISM: Impaired function of the gonads (ovaries in women and testes in men), resulting in insufficient sex hormone production.

JUVENILE CHRONIC ARTHRITIS: Chronic disease occurring in people younger than 16 years and leading to rheumatisms. Its symptoms include pain and joint swelling, as well as movement limitations.

KYPHOSIS: Concave curvature of the vertebral column which appears as a forward rounding of the back.

LEGUMES: Category of vegetables which comprises all legume seeds, including lentils, peas, beans, and soy.

MONOUNSATURATED FATTY ACIDS: Type of fatty acids which is rich in oleic acid and found in vegetable oils (olive, rapeseed, or walnut oil), goose and duck fat, and avocado.

OSTEOBLASTS: Cells responsible for bone formation and renewal.

OSTEOCLASTS: Cells responsible for bone resorption.

pH: Measure of the acidity or alkalinity of a solution, which is expressed as the power (p) of a solution to release hydrogen ions (H). pH varies between 0 and 14, with 0 being the most acidic and 14 the most alkaline. A pH above 7 is referred to as alkaline, whereas under 7, pH is acidic.

PHYTOESTROGENS: Compounds that are found in certain plants, such as soy and algae, and mimic the activity of female natural estrogen hormones.

POLYPHENOLS: Group of chemical substances contained in specific plants (fruits, vegetables, green tea, etc). They exert anti-inflammatory and antioxidant effects.

PROTEIN: Molecule composed of a long chain of amino acids. Proteins taken on a wide range of within and outside of the cells.

PROTEIN ELECTROPHORESIS: Laboratory test which consists in separating serum proteins in five fractions, i.e. albumin and other globulins. When performed in the setting of osteoporosis, this examination allows to detect conditions possibly underlying osteoporosis, such as liver cirrhosis.

RHEUMATOID POLYARTHRITIS: Chronic disease characterized by inflammatory joint manifestations. It is associated with joint pain and deformations, leading to movement restrictions.

TRACE ELEMENTS: Substances that are present in very small amounts in the body but are essential to its functioning. Trace elements bind to proteins and modify their action. As the body is unable to produce them naturally, they must be supplied by food.

ABBREVIATIONS

BMD = Bone mineral density

BMI = Body mass index

CT = Computed tomography

DEXA = Double energy X-ray absorptiometry

DHA = Docosahexaenoic acid

EPA = Eicosapentaenoic acid

HRT = Hormone replacement therapy

IU = International unit

MRI = Magnetic resonance imaging

PRAL = Potential renal acid load

SD = Standard deviation

TBS = Trabecular bone score

WHO = World Health Organization

BIBLIOGRAPHY

Book

Lane Nancy E: The osteoporosis book: A guide for patients and their families. Oxford University Press, 2001.

Sanson G: The myth of osteoporosis. MCD Century Publications, 2003.

Daniels D: Exercices for osteoporosis. Healthy Living Books, 2005.

Kessler G, Kapklein M: The bone density diet: 6 weeks to a strong body and mind. Ballantine Books, 2000.

Brown Susan E, Trivieri L: The acid-alkaline food guide: A quick reference to foods & their effect on pH levels. Square one publishers, 2006.

McCormick RK. The whole-body approach to osteoporosis: How to improve bone strength and reduce your fracture risk. New Harbinger Publications, 2009.

Publications

Remer T, Manz F. Potential Renal Acid Load of Foods and its Influence on Urine pH. J Am Diet Assoc. 1995;95:791-7.

Kok C, Sambrook PN. Secondary osteoporosis in patients with an osteoporotic fracture. Best Pract Res Clin Rheumatol 2009;23:769-79.

Verhaar HJ. Medical treatment of osteoporosis in the elderly. Aging Clin Exp Res 2009;21:407-13.

Bautmans I, Van Arkens J, Van Mackelenberg M, et al. Rehabilitation using manual mobilization for thoracic kyphosis in elderly postmenopausal patients with osteoporosis. J Rehabil Med 2010;42:129-35.

Shepherd AJ, Cass AR, Ray L. Determining risk of vertebral osteoporosis in men: validation of the male osteoporosis risk estimation score. J Am Board Fam Med 2010;23:186-94.

Guggenbuhl P. Osteoporosis in males and females: Is there really a difference? Joint Bone Spine 2009;76:595-601.

Williams GR. Actions of thyroid hormones in bone. Endokrynol Pol 2009;60:380-8.

Maggio M, Artoni A, Lauretani F, et al. The impact of omega-3 fatty acids on osteoporosis. Curr Pharm Des 2009;15:4157-64.

Tucker KL. Osteoporosis prevention and nutrition. Curr Osteoporos Rep 2009;7:111-7.

Useful information

National Osteoporosis Foundation:

http://www.nof.org/

International Osteoporosis Foundation (IOF) :

http://www.iofbonehealth.org/

In our collection Alpen éditions:

-Osteoarthrisis, Rheumatism, Arthritis

-Osteoporosis

-Control your acidity, the acid/base diet

-Handle your menopause

-The Omega-3 Answer

-Living with a Hyperactive Child

-All About the Prostate

-The French Paradox

-The XXL Syndrome

with Michel Montignac:

-The French GI Diet for Women

-Eat Yourself Slim

-The Montignac Diet Cookbook

-The French GI Diet

-Glycemic Index Diet

www.alpen.mc